MICRO-ORGANISMS
IN RUMINANT NUTRITION

Cover design
Cover drawings were kindly supplied by Monte J. Gardenier and incorporate a
photomicrograph of the anaerobic fungus *Neocallimastix*

Commission of the European Communities

Micro-organisms in Ruminant Nutrition

Edited by R.A. Prins and C.S. Stewart

A seminar in the EU programme of co-ordination of agricultural research on anaerobic fungi and their role in the nutrition of extensively fed ruminants.

DeBron Conference Centre, Dalfsen, The Netherlands
13–15 October 1993

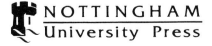
NOTTINGHAM
University Press

Nottingham University Press
Thrumpton
Nottingham NG11 0AX

NOTTINGHAM

First published 1994

British Library Cataloguing in Publication Data
Micro-organisms in Ruminant Nutrition
R.A. Prins
C.S. Stewart
A catalogue record for this book is available from the British Library

ISBN 1–897676–549

Typeset by Create Publishing Services Ltd, Bath, Avon
Printed and bound by Redwood Books, Trowbridge, Wiltshire

PREFACE

This publication contains the proceedings of a seminar 'Anaerobic fungi and their role in the nutrition of extensively fed ruminants' held in Dalfsen, the Netherlands on October 13–15, 1993 under the auspices of the Commission of European Communities programme on Agriculture.

The anaerobic fungi are the most recently discovered group of microorganisms that inhabit the rumen. Readily cultivable in the laboratory, they are implicated in the digestion of lignocellulosic components of the ruminant diet, and in the production of hydrogen which is converted to methane by methanogenic organisms. This combination of properties places the fungi at an important metabolic crossroads in the rumen fermentation; understanding the role of the rumen fungi should increase our ability to control or manipulate the rumen fermentation and its main products.

After considering the plant resources available for ruminant feeds in Europe, the characteristics of the rumen fermentation and the role of bacteria and protozoa was briefly reviewed prior to detailed examination of the life cycle, ecology and biochemical properties of the fungi. Particular emphasis was placed on ecological relationships with other rumen microorganisms, fungal enzymes involved in fibre digestion and their molecular biology, and on the function of the hydrogen-producing organelles, the hydrogenosomes. The energy metabolism, biology and possible origins of these organelles were considered in an attempt to gain fresh insights into their physiological functions. Where information on anaerobic fungi is incomplete or lacking, such as the nature of the cell-wall polymers other than chitin and the origins, function and genetics of hydrogenosomes, the characteristics of related components in other fungi, or in yeasts and protozoa, were considered as an indication of the directions in which research on anaerobic fungi should go in future.

Finally, a short discussion was held to discuss future research priorities in view of the benefits likely to accrue from increased understanding of the functions of these fascinating microorganisms.

ACKNOWLEDGEMENTS

The authors are very grateful to Mrs V. E. Smith for her invaluable secretarial help.

CONTENTS

Preface   v

1 Fibrous crops and residues for animal production in Europe   1
J. M. Abreu

2 Plant-animal and microbial interactions in ruminant   13
fibre degradation
C.S. Stewart

3 Phenolic acid composition in supernatant fluid after digestion   29
of cell walls of maize by rumen microorganisms *in vitro*:
variation between maize genotypes.
H.J.P. Marvin, C.F. Krechting, E.N. van Loo, A. Lommen,
and O. Dolstra

4 Microbial and chemical characterization of rumen contents   43
of grazing dairy cows
F. Martillotti, S. Terramoccia, C. Tripaldi, S. Puppo and
V. Danese

5 Degradation of plant cell wall polysaccharides by rumen   49
bacteria
H.J. Flint

6 Plant cell-wall degradation by rumen protozoa   69
J.P. Jouany and K. Ushida

7 Anaerobic fungi, their distribution and life cycle   79
A.P.J. Trinci, A. Rickers, K. Gull, D.R. Davies,
B.B. Nielsen, W.Y. Zhu and M.K. Theodorou

8 Plant cell wall degradation by anaerobic fungi   97
G. Fonty and PH. Gouet

9 Production of depolymerizing enzymes by anaerobic fungi   113
H.J.M. Op den Camp, R. Dijkerman, M.J. Teunissen and
C. van der Drift

10   The xylanolytic system of rumen anaerobic fungi   127
B. Gomez de Segura, R. Durand, C. Rascle, C. Fisseux
and M. Fevre

11   Cloning and expression of genes encoding enzymes of   137
the glycolytic pathway in *Neocallimastix frontalis*
R. Durand, P. Reymond-Cotton, M. Fischer, C. Rascle
and M. Fevre

12   Water-soluble polysaccharides of fungal cell walls   153
J.A. Leal

13   Cell wall composition and detection of anaerobic rumen   167
. fungi *in vivo* using fluorescent lectins
A. Breton, M. Dusser, B. Gaillard-Martinie and J. Guillot

14   Hydrogenosomes of the anaerobic fungus *Neocallimastix*   179
sp. L2.
R.A. Prins, F.D. Marvin-Sikkema, M. van der Giezen and
J.C. Gottschal

15   The evolutionary origin of hydrogenosomes from anaerobic   195
fungi
M. van der Giezen, J.C. Gottschal and R.A. Prins

16   Hydrogenosomes in anaerobic protozoa versus anaerobic   209
fungi
S. Brul and G.D. Vogels

17   Biogenesis and function of hydrogenosomes in the anaerobic   223
fungus *Neocallimastix* sp. L2; a molecular approach
W. Harder and M. Veenhuis

Overview and recommendations   233

List of participants   237

Index   245

1

FIBROUS CROPS AND RESIDUES FOR ANIMAL PRODUCTION IN EUROPE

J.M. ABREU
Instituto Superior de Agronomia, Lisboa, Portugal

Summary

This presentation gives an overview of the place of fibrous crops and residues for animal feeding in Europe (EC_{12}). The main points considered are the following:

- How much fibrous feeds (crops and residues) are produced in the EC?
- To what extent are they actually being fed to animals now?
- What is the nutritive value of these feeds?
- What, if any, are the limitations to their use in animal feeding?
- What can we do to take better advantage of these feeds in animal nutrition?

Introduction

Some preliminary remarks should be made on the data contained in this paper. The fundamental point not to be forgotten is that the figures presented should be taken only as broad estimates of the actual values (a) because of the very scarce and somewhat heterogeneous nature of the statistical data available for forages and fibrous residues, and (b) because when considering the EC as a whole it is necessary to talk about average values which may be meaningless in specific situations. Furthermore, it has sometimes been necessary to base calculations on data pertaining to different, albeit proximal, years.

The statistics available for the main products, and average values for the by-product : main product ratios have been used to obtain an

1

Table 1.1   STRAW:GRAIN RATIOS IN EC CONDITIONS (ADAPTED FROM 7)

Crop	Ratio	Crop	Ratio
Wheat	1.1	Pulses	3.5
Maize	1.5	Oilseeds	3.5
Barley	1.2	Roots	0.2[1]
Oats	1.3		
Rye	1.4		
Rice	1.3		
Triticale	1.3		

[1] Leaves : Roots ratio

estimate of fibrous crop residues (Table 1.1). In the case of cereals, for example, average values for the straw : grain ratio in each species have been used. Only on-farm residues were considered in this study – other fibrous residues that do not directly come out of farms, such as cereal brans and legume pods, were ignored. Tree leaves and other kinds of fibrous feeds of tree and shrub origin were ignored although these may be a useful source of nutrients in particular situations (sheep and goat feeding in Mediterranean countries, for example).

To obtain estimates for pastures and forages, calculations were based on the total area they occupy in the EC and on estimates of their dry matter (DM) production per hectare (Table 1.2).

Land use in the EC

The place that the relevant crops occupy in the European agriculture is summarized in Tables 1.3 and 1.4.

It can be concluded that:

- The agriculturally-used area (AUA) represents almost 60% of the total area (TA);

Table 1.2   AVERAGE DRY MATTER PRODUCTION OF FORAGES AND PASTURES IN THE EC (ESTIMATES, IN t/ha)

Forages	t/ha	Pastures	t/ha
Annual green fodder	7	Temporary grasses &	
Green maize	15	grazings	8
Perennial green fodder	7	Permanent grassland	6
Clover	7	Permanent meadows	7
Lucerne	12		
Others	7		

Table 1.3   CROP HARVESTED AREAS IN EC (AVERAGES FOR THE PERIOD 1989–1992) (1000 ha)

	Cereals (incl. rice)	Dried pulses	Oilseeds	Root crops	Other crops	Fodder	Pastures
EUR$_{12}$*	35,187	1,870	5,623	3,924	354	18,528	62,625
Belgium	328	4	15	172	12	325	856
Denmark	1,585	115	244	206	1	361	467
Germany	5,535	60	789	807	47	3,693	7,211
Greece	1,454	37	311	97	81	66	1,789
Spain	7,621	313	1,284	524	28	1,593	7,989
France	9,180	701	1,838	828	77	7,202	17,342
Ireland	400	2	10	70	2	1	5,775
Italy	4,389	150	620	429	96	3,088	5,836
Luxembourg	32	1	2	1	:	27	105
Netherlands	191	17	11	303	5	452	1,098
Portugal	841	256	65	121	2	120	761
United Kingdom	3,631	215	435	365	5	1,600	13,357

Based on (5) (2); (*) total harvested areas including estimated values; (:) Data not available.

- The area dedicated to pastures and fodder crops amounts to about 60% of the AUA;
- Cereals are very important crops, occupying about 30% of the AUA;
- Other crops (oilseeds and dried pulses included) are of minor relative importance, in terms of area.

How much fibrous feeds are produced in the EC?

Estimates of fibrous feeds production are presented in Tables 1.5 and 1.6.

Table 1.4   LAND USE IN EC (1000 ha)*

		% TA	% AUA
Total area (TA)	225,987	100	—
Agriculture used area (AUA)	128,080	56.7	100
Pasture and fodder	81,153	35.9	63.4
Cereals	35,187	15.6	27.5
Oilseeds	5,623	2.5	4.4
Root crops	3,924	1.7	3.1
Dried pulses	1,870	0.8	1.5
Others	357	0.0	0.0

*Reported to 1990
Sources (2, 5.)

Table 1.5 TOTAL PRODUCTION OF CEREAL, PULSE, OILSEED, ROOT AND OTHER CROP BY-PRODUCTS IN THE EC (1,000 t; BASED ON EUROSTAT AND ESTIMATES OF TABLE 1)

Crop	Production	Crop	Production
Wheat & Spelt	92,269	Dried pulses	19,258
Maize (grain)	40,055	Oilseeds	116,453
Barley	56,240	Roots	39,242
Oats & mixed grain	6,050	Other crops	531
Rye & Triticale	6,970		
Rice	2,765		

Table 1.6 TOTAL FORAGE AND PASTURE DRY MATTER PRODUCTION IN THE EC (BASED ON EUROSTAT (5) AND ESTIMATES OF TABLE 2)

Forages	1,000 t	Pastures	1,000 t
Annual green fodder	44,864	Temporary grasses & grazing	38,648
Green maize	53,756	Permanent grassland	289,004
Perennial green fodder	51,381	Permanent meadows	67,390
Lucerne	9,849		
Clover and others	2,617		
Total	161,840	Total	395,041

DM production from pastures (of which 70% corresponds to permanent grasslands) is about 395×10^6 t, thus corresponding to almost 40% of the total DM of fibrous feeds available (approximately 950×10^6 t). DM from green fodders (forages) is considerably lower, about 160×10^6 t, corresponding to less than 20% of the total. The remaining 40% corresponds to straws, roots, and other fibrous feeds.

It should be noted that green maize already occupies the first place of forages, with about 30% of the total forage DM, and its importance seems to be still increasing. DM from roots (beets, etc.) and "other crops" is of minor quantitative importance.

DM production from straws is relatively important, their total DM being of the same magnitude as the DM from pastures. But although their quantities are similar, the nutrients they provide certainly are not, the DM from straws being of much lower nutritive value than the DM from pastures.

The global figure for straws includes very different materials: cereal straws (about 60% of the straws, wheat straw being the most important), oilseed straws (more than 30% of the total), and legume straws (of minor importance). When estimating the percentage of DM of straws consumed by animals it was considered that only cereal and legume straws are consumed in significant amounts, and that cereal straws have several alternative uses.

To what extent are fibrous feeds being fed to animals?

Estimating the part of forages and residues which is actually eaten by animals is an almost impossible task; nevertheless, based on some published data and personal experience, the best estimates arrived at are summarized in Table 1.7. To check these estimates, it was considered that the average heads of cattle and sheep/goats eat about 10 kg and 1.2 kg of fibrous feed DM per day, respectively; multiplying these figures for the total cattle and sheep/goats populations in the EC, an estimate is thus obtained of the global fibrous feed consumption by animals in the EC (cattle and sheep/goats populations as published by Eurostat, for December 1990) – see Table 1.8.

The first estimate of total fibrous feeds DM consumption by animals gave an appoximate figure of 408×10^6t; the checking estimation, based on animal populations, gave an approximate figure of 341×10^6 t. The fact that two different estimates are in good agreement, suggests that the estimates should be broadly correct.

Based on all the data and estimates described so far it is concluded that of a total of more than 900 Mt fibrous feeds DM a little less than one half, about 350–400 Mt, is actually eaten by animals. Thus, more than half of the fibrous feed DM that could be used in animal feeding in EC is either lost or used for other ends; and, of the 528×10^6 t DM not consumed by animals more than half is straw!

Table 1.7   PRODUCTION AND INTAKE OF FIBROUS CROPS AND RESIDUES IN EC, BASED ON TABLE 5 AND 6 AND OUR OWN ESTIMATES (1,000 t, UNLESS OTHERWISE[1]

	Dry matter production	*Part of available feed consumed by animals (estimates) (%)*	*Dry matter consumed by animals*	*Quantities not consumed*
Straws	340,060	20	68,012	272,048
Roots	39,292	75	29,469	9,823
Other crops	531	10	53	478
Forages	161,840	70	113,288	48,552
Pastures	395,041	50	197,520	197,520
Total	936,764		408,342 (43.6%)	528,421 (56.4%)

(1) Forest and shrub materials not included.

Table 1.8   TOTAL DM FIBROUS FEEDS CONSUMED
YEARLY, BY CATTLE, SHEEP AND GOATS IN THE EC (1,000 t).

Country	DM consumed by cattle	DM consumed by sheep and goats
Belgium	11,538	64
Denmark	8,180	49
Germany	53,243	812
Greece	2,507	7,038
Spain	18,253	12,718
France	78,475	5,317
Ireland	22,006	2,628
Italy	30,058	5,320
Luxembourg	785	3
Netherlands	17,629	854
Portugal	4,894	1,847
United Kingdom	43,237	13,169
Total	290,805	49,819

Based on the cattle, sheep and goats populations (Eurostat figures for
December 1990) and average daily DM consumptions from fibrous feeds of
10 kg and 1.2 for cattle and sheep/goats, respectively.

What is the nutritive value of these feeds?

A common characteristic of these feeds is their high content of cell
walls. Their energy value is, consequently, very dependent on the rate
and extent of fibre degradation in the rumen. Because rumen metabolism of plant cell walls is the central theme of this meeting, particular attention shall be given to the content and nature of these cell
walls.

CEREAL, PULSE AND OILSEED STRAWS

Basic data on the chemical composition and nutritive value of these
feeds are presented in Tables 1.9 and 1.10. These tables show the range
of values that one can find in literature relevant for EC conditions.
    Practically all straws examined (cereal pulse and oilseed straws)
show levels of ash between 40–90 g per kg DM. (Those of rice and
sunflower are exceptions, which show very high values of 160 and
140 g kg^{-1} DM, respectively in some samples.
    Crude protein values are lowest in cereal straws (35–65 g kg^{-1} DM).
    All straws show very high values of crude fibre, usually about 40%,

Table 1.9   CHEMICAL COMPOSITION, ORGANIC MATTER DIGESTIBILITY (OMD) AND INTAKE OF CEREAL, PULSE AND OILSEED STRAWS: AVERAGE VALUES CONCERNING EC CONDITIONS (g kg[-1] DM, UNLESS OTHERWISE STATED)[1]

	DM	Ash[2]	CP	CF	OMD	Intake[3]
Cereal straws[4]	850–900	35–90	33–35	390–470	40–50	28–55
Rice straw	790–860	80–160	40–65	370–440	47–52	45–55
Maize straw	820–890	60–90	45–60	360–410	50–55	45–60
Pulse straw[5]	790–900	40–100	60–120	350–510	43–55	45–70
Oilseed straws[6]	800–930	60–140	42–105	320–520	32–60	25–60

[1]Values in this Table reflect information by many authors concerning EC conditions, including our own (except intake values, which were based exclusively on our own data); [2]Higher values are probably a consequence of soil contamination of the samples; [3]Measured with rams in metabolic cages; [4]Including wheat, barley, oats and rye straws; [5]Including horse bean, pea, lupin and lentil straws; [6]Including rape, soya bean and sunflower straws.

or higher. Sunflower (and some peas) straw show lower CF values (320–370 g kg^{-1} DM).

OM digestibility of straws is generally low, about 40 to 50% in cereals, (excepting maize) and slightly higher in legumes (about 5 points higher). Rape straw shows even lower values (32–39%), sunflower straw shows the highest (55–60%).

The intake values show the same trend; although low, they are higher in legume than in cereal straws (45–70 $vs.$ 30–60 g DM/kg $W^{0.75}$). Again rape straw differs from the others, by showing very low intake values (25–35 g DM/kg $W^{0.75}$), whereas in pea and lentil straws intake exceeds 60 g DM/kg $W^{0.75}$.

Cell wall content in cereal straws is about 750–800 g kg^{-1} DM or higher, especially in the case of wheat. Maize shows the lowest values (about 700 g kg^{-1} DM). Cellulose contents represent about 50%, hemicellulose 36 to 39% and lignin 9 to 11% of the cell wall dry matter.

Pulses straw show somewhat lower amounts of cell wall, usually 5 to

Table 1.10   CELL WALL COMPOSITION OF CEREAL, PULSE AND OILSEED STRAWS: AVERAGE VALUES CONCERNING EC CONDITIONS (g kg[-1] DM)[1]

	Cell walls	Cellulose	Hemicellulose	Lignin
Cereal straws[2]	750–820	385–435	272–293	55–92
Pulse straws[3]	580–776	321–484	169–215	83–130
Oilseed straws[4]	670–770	429–495	156–167	85–108

[1]Values in this Table reflect information by many authors concerning EC conditions, including our own; [2]Including wheat, barley, oats and rice straws; [3]Including horse bean, pea, vetch, lupin and lentil straws; [4]Including rape and sunflower straws.

10 units less than cereal straws; but vetches, sunflower and pea straws have still lower values of cell walls.

Pulse and oilseed straws have higher values of cellulose (about 60%) and of lignin (13–19%) in cell walls than cereal straws; their hemicellulose values, on the other hand, are much lower (only 20–30%).

FORAGES AND PASTURES

The composition of animal feeds, and especially the composition of pastures and forages, can vary considerably. The composition of pastures, for example, vary with species composition, place, weather, and time of the year. When attempting to describe the composition of pastures and forages we opted to present ranges of values available (many from our personal work) instead of straight averages and detailed analyses of variation. In all cases the values apply to the stage when the plants are normally eaten by animals.

Table 1.11 shows large differences in chemical composition, nutritive value and intake among different forages and pastures.

DM contents vary from 110–130 g kg^{-1} in the young plants to 300–350 g kg^{-1} in the older ones.

Ash contents are most often between 70 and 140 g kg^{-1} DM, but some lower values are observed, for example in green maize, and some higher ones too, in some young legumes and in soiled forages.

Table 1.11   CHEMICAL COMPOSITION, DIGESTIBILITY AND INTAKE OF FORAGES AND PASTURES; TYPICAL VALUES DURING THE CUTTING/GRAZING PHASES (g kg^{-1} DM UNLESS OTHERWISE STATED)[1].

	Dry matter (g kg^{-1})	Ash[2]	Crude protein	Crude fibre	Organic matter digestibility (%)	Intake g/kg $W^{0.75}$[3]
Annual green fodder						
Grasses (fresh)	150–300	60–130	80–210	210–350	60–78	55–85
Legumes (fresh)	130–300	70–150	120–230	170–320	65–80	60–95
Green maize	170–350	40–70	70–100	170–280	68–73	45–60
Lucerne	130–260	90–140	160–280	210–350	60–75	55–75
Temporary grasses and permanent grassland	110–280	70–140	100–220	190–370	55–80	55–90

[1]Values in this Table reflect information by many authors concerning EC conditions, including our own (except intake values, which were based on our own); [2]Higher values are probably a consequence of soil contamination of the samples; [3]Measured with rams in metabolic cages.

It is well known that protein content decreases with age (from 230–250 to 80–100 g kg^{-1} DM), and that for the same development phase it is lower in grasses than in legumes.

The opposite occurs with crude fibre contents, that range from 190–210 g kg^{-1} DM in the beginning to 300–350 g kg^{-1} DM at the end of the cycle (lower values for legumes, higher values for grasses).

Differences in cell wall fractions are shown in Table 1.12. Grasses have higher cell wall contents than legumes, which is mainly due to their higher hemicellulose content; their lignin contents, on the contrary, are lower.

DM digestibility also varies within wide limits, the higher values (about 80%) corresponding to the younger plants, and the lower ones (about 55–60%) corresponding to those at the end of the cycle.

The amounts ingested (determined with caged rams) follow a parallel pattern, ranging from 85–90 to 45–50 g/kg W$^{0.75}$; if we had instead used producing animals the variation would have been much higher.

What, if any, are the limitations to the use of fibrous feeds in animal feeding?

Low nutritive value and reduced intake together limit the utilization of fibrous feeds in animal production systems, especially in the more intensive ones. Apart from these technical limitations, there are also strong economical limitations: modern intensive methods of cereal production allow for low-cost production of feed grains, making it difficult for low-quality feeds such as straw to be economically fed to animals.

Table 1.12 CELL WALL COMPOSITION OF FORAGE AND PASTURES:TYPICAL VALUES DURING THE CUTTING/GRAZING PHASES (g kg^{-1} DM).[1][2]

	Cellulose	*Hemicellulose*	*Lignin*
Annual green fodder			
Grasses (fresh)	26–35	18–25	3–7
Legumes (fresh)	20–32	8–11	4–9
Green maize	21–29	20–22	3–6
Lucerne	19–30	10–12	7–11
Temporary grasses and permanent grassland	23–33	14–27	4–9

[1]Cellulose as ADF-ADL, Hemicellulose as NDF-ADF and Lignin as ADL (7); DM = Dry matter; [2]Values in this Table reflect information by many authors concerning EC conditions, including our own (except intake values, which were based exclusively on our own data).

The increasing specialization of farms is another factor that can limit the use of fibrous feeds, because (1) animals, being separated from fibrous feeds, cannot consume them locally, and (2) transporting these products over long distances is usually uneconomical.

The low digestibility of fibrous feeds – about one half of the organic matter ingested is excreted in the faeces – can be another disadvantage in situations where waste disposal problems are important.

Whenever there are alternative uses for fibrous products less of them may be available for animal feeding.

It is not uncommon for fibrous feeds to contain toxic or anti-nutritional factors (4), requiring care in their administration to animals. Although some of these factors can be reduced or eliminated by plant breeding, new varieties obtained are often less resistant to pests and diseases; one alternative hypothesis is to eliminate or inactivate them through chemical or other treatments (there are even cases when the toxic factors, once extracted, can be put to good use).

What can we do to take better advantage of these feeds in animal feeding?

It seems that less than half the fibrous feeds in the EC are eaten by animals (their use can of course be higher in some regions). It can logically be concluded that there should be opportunities for increasing and improving the use of these feeds.

In the case of pastures, particular attention should be given to plant and animal management; in the case of forages great importance should be given to adequate cutting times and methods of conservation.

By-products in some cases would be better utilized after physical, chemical and microbiological treatments. Improved conditions for rumen fermentation and animals selected for better intakes also ought to be considered.

References and further reading

(1)   ABREU, J., CALOURO, M. and SOARES, A. (1982). Tabelas de Valor Alimentar – Forragens Mediterranicas Cultivadas em Portugal – 1ª contribuicao. ISA, Lisboa.
(2)   COMISSAO DAS COMUNIDADES EUROPEIAS, (1992). A

situacao da Agricultura na Comunidade, Relatorio, 1992. Servico das Publicacoes Oficiais das Comunidades Europeias, Luxemburgo.

(3)   DE BOER, F. and BICKEL, H. (Eds), (1988). Livestock feed resources and feed evaluation in Europe – Present situation and future prospects. Elsevier. Amsterdam.

(4)   DUFFUS, C.M. and DUFFUS, H.J. (1991). Introduction and overview. In: J. P. D'Mello, C.M., Duffus and J.H. Duffus (Eds): Toxic substances in crop plants. The Royal Society of Chemistry, Cambridge, U.K.

(5)   EUROSTAT, (1993). Crop production – Quarterly statistics, 1993 (2). Statistical Office of European Communities, Luxembourg.

(6)   KOSSILA, V.L. (1984). Location and potential field use. In Straw and other fibrous by-products as feed. Sundstol, F. and Owen, E. (Eds), pp 4–24 Elsevier. Amsterdam.

(7)   ROBERTSON, J.B. and VAN SOEST, P.J. (1981). In The Analysis of Dietary Fiber. James, W.P.T. and Theander, O. (Eds): Marcel Dekker, New York.

(8)   THOMAS, C. and CHAMBERLAIN, D.G. (1990). Evaluation and prediction of the nutritive value of pastures and forages. In Feedstuff Evaluation. J. Wiseman and D.J. Cole (Eds.): Butterworths, Cambridge, U.K.

2

PLANT-ANIMAL AND MICROBIAL INTERACTIONS IN RUMINANT FIBRE DEGRADATION

C.S. STEWART

Rowett Research Institute, Bucksburn, Aberdeen, AB2 9SB, UK.

Summary

The nutritional performance of grazing and browsing ruminants depends on complex interactions between plants, animals and the rumen microorganisms. Forage intake is influenced by plant type and maturity, and by climatic conditions. The anatomical features of plants affect their rate of fermentation and fragmentation and these factors affect degradation by determining the time for which the plant material is exposed to the microorganisms in the rumen. Some plants, especially forage legumes, possess toxic secondary metabolites and the rumen microbial transformation of these toxins offers prospects for increasing the utilization of such plants for animal production. Important microbe-microbe interactions include predation, interspecies cross-feeding and amensalism. Amensalistic interactions, because they involve the inhibition of some microorganisms by factors produced by others, are of particular interest because we may eventually be able to use the knowledge gained from the study of microbial inhibitors to control the species composition and activity of the rumen microbial flora.

Introduction to forage degradability

Forage degradability is affected by plant, animal and environmental factors. Large animals are in general capable of more extensive degradation of forage than are small animals; here, the controlling factor is probably the time for which plant material is exposed to the gut microbial population. The higher intake and faster rate of digestion of

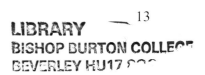

legume forages compared to grasses is most commonly attributed to the more rapid fragmentation of legumes in the rumen; this process increases the surface area exposed for microbial colonization and speeds passage through the gut. Increasing plant maturity is usually accompanied by decreased intake and degradability, presumably as a consequence of increased lignification and recalcitrance. Feed supplements may be used to increase the metabolizable energy or nitrogen content of the diet; such supplements affect the fermentation of fibre in different ways. Supplementary grain may decrease forage intake and degradability, partly as a result of lowered rumen pH (32), but also possibly as a result of the repression or inhibition of cellulolysis. In contrast, protein supplements tend to increase the intake of poor quality forages. Processing that reduces the size of feed particles tends to increase feed intake and possibly also the rate of ruminal fermentation, but may decrease the extent of degradation by decreasing the rumen residence time. Cold stress increases rumen motility and digesta passage, leading to increased feed intake. Conversely, heat stress tends to result in decreased intake which may increase fibre degradation by increasing the rumen residence time (reviewed in 13).

Toxic constituents of plants

Many plant possess toxic components which reduce their susceptibility to predation by animals. Perhaps the most significant example in ruminant nutrition is that of the non-proteic amino acid mimosine, found in the leaves of the legume *Leucaena leucocephala*. In Australia, *Leucaena* was toxic to ruminants until rumen bacteria, capable of degrading mimosine and its toxic products, were introduced from Hawaii and Indonesia. It is now known than mimosine and its toxic derivatives can be degraded by several types of bacteria, including *Synergistes jonesii* (1), at least one *Clostridium* species and other, so far unidentified, strains (10,12). It seems that the rumen flora shows at least some geographical variation. This has led to increased interest in the nature of plant toxic factors and their microbial detoxification. In particular, experiments are in progress to develop genetically engineered strains capable of the anaerobic degradation of the toxin fluoroacetate, a component of some *Gastrolobium* and *Oxylobium* species (14), and bacteria capable of transforming other potentially toxic plant components are being sought (11). Other plant components may inhibit the fementation of plant material in the rumen. The inhibition of rumen (carboxy-methyl)cellulase by a water-soluble extract from the forage sericea has been described (31). The inhibition was suppressed by treatment of the extracts with polyphenol oxidase, implicating a polyphenolic compound. Phenolics, tannins and leucoanthocyanins were assumed to be responsible for the inhibition of pectinases by extracts from fruit and from the leaves of grape and other plants (22). Of the 212 samples of fresh leaves, flowers fruit and seeds tested, significant inhibitory activity towards the cellulase of the aerobic fungus *Trichoderma* was detected in 41 (22). Prominent among the plants which contained cellulase inhibitors were the leaves of bayberry (*Myrica pensylvanica*), muscadine grape (*Vitis rotundifolia*), *Vaccinium nitidum*, *Comptonia peregrina*, *Lespedeza cuneata* and *Diospyros virginiana*. Further investigation of the bayberry inhibitor showed that it was able to bind readily to proteins and that it acted as a non-competitive enzyme inhibitor. Several natural tannins and the lower MW phenols haematoxylin, 3-5-4' trihydroxystilbene and its glucoside, pyrogallol and tannic acid were also shown to inhibit *Trichoderma* cellulase.

In many arid, semi-arid and cold mountainous areas, the leaves of trees and shrubs are fed to ruminants either fresh, or after drying. Normally, tree leaves and browse contain both condensed and hydrolysable tannins (39). Tannins depress intake by a variety of mechanisms, and have been shown to depress fermentation, reduce wool growth, decrease nutrient availablity (especially sulphur) and cause toxicity in ruminants and other animals. Tannins form precipitates with proteins, and inhibit many enzyme reactions non-specifically. Microbial enzymes inhibited by tannins from *Quercus incana* include urease, carboxymethyl cellulase, glutamate dehydrogenase and alanine aminotransferases. Curiously, the activity of glutamate ammonia ligase in the rumen was increased in the presence of *Quercus* tannins. Tannins from *Robinia* were shown to inhibit β-glucosidase activity, and tannins from *Ziziphus* inhibited casein hydrolysis (20).

The plant phenolics p-coumaric and ferulic acid inhibit growth and cellulolysis by rumen bacteria in pure culture (8). Coumarin (1,2 benzopyrone) inhibits glucose fermentation by rumen anaerobic fungi (5). Although these compounds were tested at concentrations greater than would be found in the bulk phase of rumen contents, their local concentration might be high in the microenvironment of the degrading plant cell wall surface (8).

Apart from the possibility of introducing rumen microorganisms capable of degrading plant toxins, identifying the toxins present in different plants is useful to plant breeders. Ruminant diets may also be

supplemented with chemicals, such as polyvinyl pyrrolidine and polyethylene glycol that form complexes with phenolics, reducing their
toxic effects.

Plant anatomy and degradation

The microbial digestion of the polymers of the plant cell wall is the
central event of forage degradation. However the anatomical organization of the tissues in which plant cells occur varies in different plants,
thus affecting their degradability. For example, marked anatomical
differences exist between legumes and grasses and between plants
which use the C_3 and C_4 photosynthetic pathways. The leaves of
legumes and C_3 grasses tend to have an open structure, with a sub-
stantial proportion of air space compared to those of typical C_4 grasses.
Indeed, the leaves of temperate legumes may be fermented so rapidly
that bloat is induced. Thin-walled plant cells tend to be degraded
without microbial adhesion, but adhesion is necessary for the degradation of thick-walled cells (6). The accessibility of sclerenchyma and
vascular tissue is limited, as the cells are held tightly together by the
lignified middle lamella. Cell disruption is required so that cellulolytic
microorganisms can gain access to the inner luminal surfaces of the
cells to effect attack. Factors that reduce the rate of tissue disintegration therefore reduce degradability. Such factors include the presence of secondary thickened (and therefore slowly degradable)
parenchyma bundle sheath cells in some C_4 grasses, the interlocking of
epidermal cells of tropical grasses, preventing easy separation (43) and
the presence in some grasses of bundles of sclerenchyma cells effectively
linking the vascular tissues with the epidermis.

Intrinsic factors limiting plant cell wall degradation

The composition and molecular arrangement of plant cell wall (CW)
polymers has been very widely reviewed (7, 18, 39). Some of the
intrinsic factors that limit the rate or extent of CW hydrolysis by rumen
microorganisms are listed in Table 2.1. The organisation of the polymers in the CW of grasses and legumes differs significantly, and these
differences affect susceptibility to degradation. Cheng and his colleagues (reviewed in 6) found that the pectinolytic rumen anaerobe
Lachnospira multiparus rapidly macerated leaflets of clover but had

Table 2.1 INTRINSIC FACTORS LIMITING PLANT CELL WALL
DEGRADATION (*WHERE NO REFERENCE IS CITED, THE TOPIC IS COVERED
IN 7, 18 AND 39)

Factor	Effect and reference*
Cellulose organization	Highly ordered forms of cellulose are attacked relatively slowly, but this is in part due to the low area: volume ratio of the substrates tested (41). Highly ordered and disordered cellulose are lost from fibre at about the same rate. Cotton-degrading forms of *Ruminococcus flavefaciens* degrade barley straw at the same rate as non-cotton degrading forms (35).
Lignification	Probably the major factor: forms a barrier, covalently attached to polysaccharides, esp. hemicellulose via ferulate-arabinose links.
Hemicellulose acetylation	Deacetylation increases susceptibility to degradation.
Low MW phenolics	Potentially inhibitory on release.
Silica	Si content and degradability inversely related.
Low N,P,S	May be limiting in low quality forages.
Particle size	Determines surface area:volume ratio, and residence time.
Others	Cutins, waxes, suberins may form inert barriers and provide mastication resistance.

no comparable effect on grasses, reflecting differences between these plants in the distribution of pectic substances, especially in the middle lamella. Other important differences exist. For example, 4-hydroxycin-namic acids are thought to cross-link glucurono-arabinoxylans to lignin in grasses, but not in legumes (15). Despite such differences and the fact that CW degradability is influenced by many intrinsic factors (Table 2.1), there is general agreement that the controlling factors in plant cell wall degradation are those that determine the access of the rumen microoganisms and their enzymes, many of which have high MW and are organized into macromolecular complexes (cellulosomes) (21), to the hydrolysable polymers. Chief among these factors are the presence of lignin covalantly bound to polysaccharides and the highly branched structure of some polymers limiting the access of microbial enzymes to susceptible bonds (15).

Modelling CW transformation in the gut

Blaxter *et al* (4) fed dried grass to sheep and showed that the passage and digestion of the grass was affected by its particle size. In particular, extending the residence time of the grass in the gut increased digestion. Later, Waldo (40) suggested that cellulose disappearance from the gut was the result of two simultaneous first-order processes, passage and digestion:

$A = A_o e^{-(k1+k2)t}$ (A = digestion & passage of the digestible component)
$B = B_o e^{-(k2)t}$ (B = passage of the indigestible component)

in which A_o = amount of potentially digestible cellulose present initially: B_o = amount of indigestible cellulose present initially: k1 = rate of digestion; k2 = rate of passage; t = time after feeding (h). Later models have incorporated a lag phase prior to attack, (a period during which bacteria attach to the plant CW) and the presence of CW which are degraded at different rates. First order kinetics has also been used to describe the disappearance of CW and other substrates from mesh bags in the rumen (reviewed in 39). The use of first order kinetics seems inappropriate in view of the insoluble and physically complex, heterogeneous nature of the CW. However, a truly mechanistic model of this complex process is bound to be difficult to achieve, and CW digestion has been argued to show essentially first order kinetics in vitro (40). Shi and Weimer (30) showed that cellulolysis by *Ruminococcus flavefaciens* in continuous culture did not follow first order kinetics at low dilution rates, but suggested that this might have been due to low rates of cellulase synthesis. Cellulolysis is limited by the presence of lignin-hemicellulose complexes preventing access of the cellulolytic organisms and/or their enzymes, so perhaps the closest approximation to reality would be to assume that cellulolysis is a pseudo-first order process subject to non-competitive inhibition. Although lignification is usually regarded as being an 'extent' rather than a rate-limiting factor, it seems likely that the very close association of the matrix polymers and the cellulose in CW must have some influence on the rate of cellulolysis. Observations on the digestion of barley straw by rumen microorganisms (6, 33) suggest that the thicker-walled cells are degraded by bacteria adherent to the inner luminal surface. Thus, during degradation, the walls become thinner, and microbial growth has to occur at a rate sufficient to maintain saturation of the gradually increasing wall surface with bacteria producing the large MW, membrane-associated enzyme complexes responsible for cellulose and hemicellulose hydrolysis. Most thick-walled plant cells are cylindrical in shape. The area (a) of the inner luminal surface of a cylinder of length l and inner radius r cm is $2\pi lr$ cm^2. The instantaneous rate of change of a for any value of r ($\delta a/\delta r\ 2\pi lr$) = $2\pi l$. How quickly r changes during degradation of thick walled tissues cells is not known, but image analysis is being used to measure the cell wall thickness, density and area, and the cell radius of tissues (epidermis, cortex, phloem vascular tissue and parenchyma) of varieties of winter oil seed rape (*Brassica napus*)(37), and this technique could also be used to estimate the relationship between degradation rate and anatomical parameters.

Plant cell wall degrading microbes and their interactions

The bacteria, fungi and protozoa that degrade CW in the rumen are described in the papers by Flint, Fonty and Gouet and by Jouany and Ushida in this volume. Fungal enzymes involved in CW degradation are described by Durand and Fevre, and the role of hydrogenosomes in cellulolytic fungi and some other prokaryotes is covered in the remaining papers. The interactions that occur between rumen microbes have been reviewed in (44) and interactions involved in fibre degradation are reviewed in (9). The relative contribution of bacteria, protozoa and fungi to CW degradation is poorly understood, and R.E. Hungate's view that 'protozoa are important when they are present' should probably be extended to other groups such as the fungi and the large, so far uncultivable, bacteria also. Some rumen ciliate protozoa such as *Polyplastron* predate on bacteria, fungal zoospores, and other protozoa such as *Entodinium* (17). Studies on defaunated and selectively refaunated ruminants have proved informative about the interactions of the protozoa. Such studies have shown that the presence of ciliate protozoa reduces the numbers of bacteria in the rumen, especially when concentrates are fed. The re-introduction of *Entodinium* sp. reduced the total numbers of viable bacteria, but did not lower the count of cellulolytic bacteria when *Polyplastron* was present. The re-introduction of *Dasytricha* depressed the numbers of all kinds of bacteria studied and had the most marked effects when roughages were fed (25). It is argued that predation by protozoa on bacteria leads to increased concentrations of nutrients like ammonia and phosphate which may relieve nutrient limitations of the surviving bacteria. The non-specific predation of bacteria by protozoa probably contributes to the species and strain diversity of the bacterial population, by operating most heavily against the numerically predominant bacteria that might otherwise swamp the system (reviewed in 25). It has recently been shown that the addition of protozoa to dense suspensions of rumen bacteria did not increase fermentation of hay and barley straw *in vitro* (16). The beneficial effects of the presence of ciliates on CW digestion seem therefore to relate to the improved nutrition of CW degrading bacteria, rather than to the provision of a CW degrading process unique to protozoa.

The presence of rumen bacteria in mixed culture with rumen fungi may result in the inhibition or stimulation of fungal cellulolytic activity, depending on the bacterial species used. Rumen fungi produce some of the most active cellulases known (Fonty and Gouet, this volume). However, some strains of *Ruminococcus albus* (26, 36) and *R. flavefaciens* (2,3,26,36) have been shown to produce soluble factors that inhibit fungal cellulolysis, but do not affect the growth of fungi on soluble sugars and have little effect on xylan utilization. Fungal cellulolysis is also reduced in the presence of several soluble sugars (galactose, mannose and fucose) and the lectins con A and SBA (34). The binding of these compounds to receptors on the fungal wall is being studied with the aim of characterizing the fungal cell surface and its role in adhesion and cellulolysis (34). Although the inhibitory activity of the ruminococci is associated with proteins, it is now known that incubation with protease does not destroy the activity of the inhibitor from *R. flavefaciens* strain 17. However, periodate treatment (to oxidize carbohydrates) has been found to abolish inhibitory activity. Chemical analysis of the inhibitor suggests that it contains lipo-teichoic acids, polymers of glycerol-, ribitol- or mannitol phosphate substituted with amino acids and/or sugars. These are components that occur in the cell envelope of many Gram positive bacteria; they are readily released into culture supernatants (42). These polyelectrolytes serve as phage receptor sites, and the lipoteichoic acids of *Streptococcus* may be involved in adhesion. It is now thought that lipo-teichoic acids or their components play a role in fungal inhibition by ruminococci, and this possibility is being investigated. Although amensalistic interactions have been reported to occur between bacteria isolated from the monogastric gut (38), this is the first example in which the growth of some rumen organisms appears to be limited by factors produced by others. If the mechanism of this effect can be clearly established, it may lead to new methods for manipulating the species composition and activity of the rumen microbial flora. It seems unlikely that such interactions are limited to the example currently under investigation, and a wide range of rumen organisms are now being screened for the production of inhibitors. In the long term it is hoped that the proliferation of 'undesirable' bacteria such as the causative agent of acidosis, *Streptococcus bovis* might be controlled if a suitable inhibitor can be found among the products of the commensal flora.

The rumen fungi produce hydrogen which is converted to methane by methanogens. Marvin-Sikkema *et al.* (23) showed that co-culture of rumen fungi with the hydrogenotrophic, saccharolytic bacterium

Selenomonas ruminantium resulted in the disappearance of hydrogen and the appearance of propionate, presumably formed by diversion of reduced cofactors to the reduction of fumarate to succinate. Richardson and Stewart (unpublished data) have shown that the addition of *S. ruminantium* to co-cultures of *Neocallimastix* sp. strain RE1 markedly reduces the accumulation of methane.

It has been supposed that the interactions between rumen CW degrading bacterial species are dominated by competition for substrate (between active CW degraders) and the cross-feeding of soluble products of cellulose hydrolysis (27). The predominant cellulolytic rumen bacteria share some nutritional requirements for growth factors (17), but this was not thought to contribute to interactions between *Ruminococcus flavefaciens* and *Fibrobacter succinogenes* growing on barley straw and clover (28). Here, it was argued that these species show less degradative activity towards clover in mixed culture than does *R. flavefaciens* in monoculture because the less rapidly acting bacterium (*F. succinogenes*) attaches to the CW and excludes the ruminococcus from parts of the substrate. The use of phospholipid markers confirmed that *F. succinogenes* was outgrown by the ruminococcus in these experiments, but the presence of *F. succinogenes* tended to lower the viable numbers of ruminococci. The fate of some of the monosaccharides released from the plant material during these incubations was also investigated, and it was clear that greater quantities of the sugars released from hemicellulose (xylose and arabinose) accumulated in culture supernatants than did glucose from cellulose. Miron and his colleagues (24) showed that soluble bound sugars from hemicellulose hydrolysis by *Fibrobacter* and *Ruminococcus* were utilized by *Butyrivibrio fibrisolvens* in mixed culture, whereas negligible cross-feeding of cellulose hydrolysis products occurred. It seems that there are several substrate pools present, including:

- insoluble but hydrolysable CW polymers (long half-life)
- soluble free sugars (very short half life)
- sugars (presumably covalently bound) in oligosaccharides, glycosides and lignin-carbohydrate complexes (LCC) (medium to long half life)

The LCC found in the rumen (7) are presumably remnants of larger complexes that are further degraded by microbes following their release from CW, and comparing the complexes released by different pure cultures could help us to understand the nature and origins of LCC. The sugar composition of the soluble products from the degradation of clover and straw by cellulolytic bacteria are similar (28) despite the differences in the composition and structure of these plants. However, when phospholipid analysis was carried out on plant material incubated in the rumen in nylon bags, clover and straw were found to be colonized by very different CW degrading populations (29).

The importance of microbial aggregation

Examination of the rumen microbial population by microscopy demonstrates the presence of mixed consortia occupying the liquid phase of the digesta, and adherent to the solids (6). By analogy with other habitats that support the growth of a mixed microbial flora, it is likely that interactions based on surface contact between the various species, or their extracellular capsules, are important in allowing those organisms that interact in a positive way (i.e. in interspecies cross-feeding) to coaggregate, forming mixed colonies (19). This would reduce distances over which nutrients involved in interspecies cross-feeding would have to diffuse. The antagonism expressed by some rumen bacteria such as the ruminococci towards the fungi may result in the failure of these organisms to coaggregate to form a stable, mixed, adherent population with the fungi. Some of these proposed interactions are illustrated schematically in Fig. 2.1.

Adaptive responses of *R. flavefaciens* to growth on CW

Mutations occur in *R. flavefaciens* during long term cultivation on different cellulosic substrates (35). Recently Saluzzi (29) has shown that during culture on ryegrass, *R. flavefaciens* strain 17 increased both total and specific xylanase activity by 3 to 4 fold; there were much smaller changes in the production of cellulases and other enzymes including arabinofuranosidases. This experiment suggests that xylanases play an important role in the degradation of ryegrass CW by whole cultures of this bacterium, and that assay of this activity might predict the CW degradative ability of these bacteria. They also suggest that mutations are likely to be important in determining the success of individual species in the rumen.

Microbial interactions in plant cell wall degradation

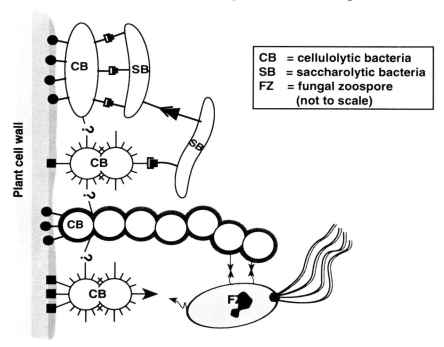

Figure 2.1. Scheme showing possible interactions between bacteria and fungi involved in fibre degradation. Co-aggregation (—[■—, —<◄—) is probably important in facilitating cross-feeding between cell-wall degrading (CB) and sugar-fermenting bacteria (SB). Interactions between cellulolytic bacteria (?) are not well understood, but presumably include competition for new attachment sites during growth. The inhibition of some anaerobic fungi (FZ) by ruminococci (—►◄—) may be due to surface components released from the bacterial cells.

Conclusions

The interactive nature of the factors affecting forage degradation by ruminants provide many means for manipulating forage degradation. The possible application of microorganisms with beneficial properties such as the ability to degrade plant toxins or the overproduction of metabolites depends on futher understanding the interactions that determine the success of particular strains. The interactions that involve the inhibition of some organisms by factors produced by others are likely to be of particular importance in offering the means to manipulate the rumen microbial flora and its activities.

Acknowledgements

C. S. Stewart is supported by the Scottish Office Agriculture and Fisheries Department.

References

(1) ALLISON, M.J., MAYBERRY, W.R., McSWEENEY, C.S. and STAHL, D.A.(1992). *Synergistes jonesii* gen. nov. sp. nov. a rumen bacterium that degrades pyridinediols. Syst. Appl. Microbiol. 15, 522–529.
(2) BERNALIER, A. (1991). Les champignons anaerobies du rumen: caracterisation et interactions avec les bacteries du rumen dans la cellulyse in vitro. PhD thesis. Universite Blaise Pascal, Clermont Ferrand, France. No. d'ordre DU 281.
(3) BERNALIER, A., FONTY, G., BONNEMAY, F. and GOUET, PH. (1993). Inhibition of the cellulolytic activity of *Neocallimastix frontalis* by *Ruminococcus flavefaciens*. J. Gen. Microbiol. 139, 873–880.
(4) BLAXTER, K.L., GRAHAM, N.McC. and WAINMAN, F.W. (1956). Some observations on the digestibility of food by sheep and on related problems. Brit. J. Nutr. 10, 69–91.
(5) CANSUNAR, E., RICHARDSON, A.J., WALLACE, G. and STEWART, C.S. (1990). Effect of coumarin on glucose uptake by anaerobic rumen fungi in the presence and absence of *Methanobrevibacter smithii*. FEMS Microbiol. Lett. 70, 157–160.
(6) CHENG, K.-J., STEWART, C.S., DINSDALE, D. and COSTERTON, J.W. (1983/84). Electron microscopy of bacteria involved in the digestion of plant cell walls. Anim. Fd Sci. Technol. 10, 39–120.
(7) CHESSON, A. (1993). Mechanistic models of forage cell wall degradation. In Forage Cell Wall Structure and Digestibility. (Jung, H.G. et al. eds) pp. 347–376. ASA, CSSA and SSSA: Madison.
(8) CHESSON, A., STEWART, C.S. and WALLACE, R.J. (1982). Influence of plant phenolic acids on growth and cellulolytic activity of rumen bacteria. Appl. Environ. Microbiol. 44, 597–603.
(9) DEHORITY, B.A. (1993). Microbial Ecology of Cell Wall Fermentation. In Forage Cell Wall Structure and Digestibility.

(Jung, H.G. et al. eds) pp.425–454. ASA, CSSA and SSSA: Madison.

(10) DOMINGUEZ-BELLO, M.G. and STEWART, C.S. (1990). Degradation of mimosine, 2,3 dihydroxypyridine and 3(hydroxy)-4-(1H)-pyridone by bacteria from the rumen of sheep in Venezuela. FEMS Microbiol. Ecol. 73, 283–290.

(11) DOMINGUEZ-BELLO, M.G. and STEWART, C.S. (1991). Effect of feeding *Canavalia ensiformis* on the rumen flora of sheep, and of the toxic amino acid canavanine on rumen bacteria. Syst. Appl. Microbiol. 13, 388–393.

(12) DOMINGUEZ-BELLO, M.G. and STEWART, C.S. (1991). Characteristics of a rumen *Clostridium* capable of degrading mimosine, 3(OH)-4-(1H)-pyridone and 2,3 dihydroxypyridone. Syst. Appl. Microbiol. 14, 67–71.

(13) GALYEAN, M.L. and GOETSCH, A.L. (1993). Utilization of forage fiber by ruminants. In Forage Cell Wall Structure and Digestibility. (Jung, H.G. et al. eds) pp. 33–72. ASA, CSSA and SSSA: Madison.

(14) GREGG, K. and SHARPE, H. (1991). Enhancement of rumen microbial detoxification by gene transfer. In Physiological Aspects of Digestion and Metabolism in Ruminants (Tsuda, T. et al. eds) pp. 719–735. Academic Press: San Diego.

(15) HATFIELD, R.D. (1993). Cell wall polysaccharide interactions and degradability. In Forage Cell Wall Structure and Digestibility. (Jung, H.G. et al. eds) pp.285–314. ASA, CSSA and SSSA: Madison.

(16) HIDAYAT, HILLMAN, K., NEWBOLD, C.J. and STEWART, C.S. (1993). The contributions of bacteria and protozoa to ruminal forage fermentation *in vitro*, as determined by microbial gas production. Anim. Fd Sci. Technol. 42, 193–208.

(17) HUNGATE, R.E. (1966). The Rumen and its Microbes. Academic Press: NY.

(18) JUNG, H.G. and DEETZ, D.A. (1993). Cell wall lignification and degradabilty. In Forage Cell Wall Structure and Digestibility. (Jung, H.G. et al. eds) pp. 315–346. ASA, CSSA and SSSA: Madison.

(19) KOLENBRANDER, P.E. and LONDON, J. (1992). Ecological significance of coaggregation among oral bacteria. In Advances in Microbial Ecology, Vol. 12. (Marshall, K.C., ed.) pp. 183–217. Plenum Press, NY.

(20) KUMAR, R. and VAITHIYANATHAN, S. (1990). Occur-

rence, nutritional significance and effect on animal productivity of tannins in tree leaves. Anim. Fd Sci. Technol. 30, 21038.

(21)   LAMED, R.L., NAIMARK, J., MORGENSTERN, E. and BAYER, E.J. (1987). Specialized cell-surface structures in cellulolytic bacteria. J. Bacteriol. 169, 3792–3800.

(22)   MANDELS, M. and REESE, E.T. (1963). Inhibition of cellulases and β-glucosidases. In Advances in Enzymic Hydrolysis of Cellulose and Related Materials (Reese, E.T. ed) pp. 115–157 Pergamon Press: Oxford.

(23)   MARVIN-SIKKEMA, F.D., RICHARDSON, A.J., STEWART, C.S., GOTTSCHAL, J.C. and PRINS, R.A. (1990). Influence of hydrogen-consuming bacteria on cellulose degradation by anaerobic fungi. Appl. Environ. Microbiol. 56, 3793–3797.

(24)   MIRON, J., DUNCAN, S.H. and STEWART, C.S. (1994). Interactions between rumen bacterial strains during the degradation and utilization of the monosaccharides of barley straw cell walls. J. Appl. Bacteriol.

(25)   PRINS, R.A. (1991). The rumen ciliates and their functions. In Rumen Microbial Metabolism and Ruminant Digestion (J.-P. Jouany, ed.) pp. 39–52. INRA: Paris.

(26)   RICHARDSON, A.J. STEWART, C.S., CAMPBELL, G.P., WILSON, A.B. and JOBLIN, K.N. (1986). Influence of co-culture with rumen bacteria on the lignocellulolytic activity of phycomycetous fungi from the rumen. Abstracts XIV International Congress of Microbiology, PG2–24, 233.

(27)   RUSSELL, J.B. (1985). Fermentation of cellodextrins by cellulolytic and non-cellulolytic rumen bacteria. Appl. Environ. Microbiol. 49, 572–576.

(28)   SALUZZI, L., SMITH, A. and STEWART, C.S. (1993). Analysis of bacterial phospholipid markers and plant monosaccharides during forage degradation by *Ruminococcus flavefaciens* and *Fibrobacter succinogenes*. J. Gen. Microbiol. 139, 2865–2873.

(29)   SALUZZI,L. (1993). Ecophysiology of cellulolytic bacteria in the rumen. PhD Thesis, University of Aberdeen.

(30)   SHI, Y. and WEIMER, P.J. (1992). Response surface analysis of the effect of pH and dilution rate on *Ruminococcus flavefaciens* FD-1 in cellulose-fed continuous culture. Appl. Environ. Microbiol. 58, 2583–2591.

(31)   SMART, W.W.G., BELL, T.A., STANLEY, N.W. and COPE,

W.A. (1961). Inhibition of rumen cellulase by an extract from *Sericea* forage. J. Dairy Sci. 44, 1945–1946.

(32) STEWART, C.S. (1977). Factors affecting the cellulolytic activity of rumen contents. Appl. Environ. Microbiol. 33, 497–502.

(33) STEWART, C.S. (1985). A summary of the OECD collaborative experiments on ammoniation of barley straw. In Improved Utilisation of Lignocellulosic Materials in Animal Feed. pp. 124–142. OECD: Paris.

(34) STEWART, C.S., DUNCAN, S.H., BEGBIE, R. and RICHARDSON, A.J. (1992). Inhibition of fungal cellulolytic activity by an extracellular protein produced by *Ruminococcus flavefaciens* strain 17. Proc. Soc. Gen. Microbiol. Glasgow, June 1992 p. 8

(35) STEWART, C.S., DUNCAN, S.H., McPHERSON, C.A. RICHARDSON, A.J. and H.J. (1990). The implications of the loss and regain of cotton-degrading activity for the degradation of straw by *Ruminococcus flavefaciens* strain 007. J. Appl. Bacteriol. 68, 349–356.

(36) STEWART, C.S., DUNCAN, S.H., RICHARDSON, A.J. BACKWELL, C. and BEGBIE, R. (1992). The inhibition of fungal cellulolysis by cell-free preparations from ruminococci. FEMS Microbiol. Lett. 97, 83–88.

(37) TRAVIS, A.J., MURISON, S.D., CHESSON, A. and WALKER, K.C. (1993). Quantitative measurement of stem anatomy as an indicator of varietal performance. In Physiology of Varieties (White, E. et al. eds) pp. 335–343. Assoc. Appl. Biol.: Wellesborne.

(38) VANDEVOORDE, L., VANDE WOESTYNE, M., BRUYNEEL, B., CHRISTIAENS, H., and VERSTRAATE, W. (1992). Critical factors governing the behaviour of lactic acid bacteria in mixed cultures. In The Lactic Acid Bacteria Volume 1. (Wood, B.J.B. ed.) pp. 447–476. London: Elsevier Applied Sciences.

(39) VAN SOEST, P.J. (1982). The Nutritional Ecology of the Ruminant. O&B Books: Corvallis.

(40) WALDO, D.R., SMITH, L.W. and COX, E.L. (1972). Model of cellulose disappearance from the rumen. J. Dairy Sci. 55, 125–129.

(41) WEIMER. P.J. LOPEZ-GUIZA, J.M. and FRENCH, A.D. (1990). Effect of cellulose fine structure on kinetics of its diges-

tion by mixed ruminal microorganisms in vitro. Appl. Environ. Microbiol. 56, 2421–2429.

(42)   WELLSTOOD, S. (1992). Gram positive cocci. In Encyclopaedia of Microbiology Vol. 2 (Lederberg, J. ed.) pp. 319–329. San Diego: Academic Press.

(43)   WILSON, J.R. (1993). Organization of forage plant tissues. In Forage Cell Wall Structure and Digestibility. (Jung, H.G. et al. eds) pp. 1–32. ASA, CSSA and SSSA: Madison.

(44)   WOLIN, M.J. and MILLER, T.L. (1988). Microbe-microbe interactions. In The Rumen Microbial Ecosystem (Hobson, P.N. ed) pp. 343–360. London: Elsevier Applied Science.

3

PHENOLIC ACID COMPOSITION IN SUPERNATANT FLUID AFTER DIGESTION OF CELL WALLS OF MAIZE BY RUMEN MICROORGANISMS *IN VITRO*: VARIATION BETWEEN MAIZE GENOTYPES.

H.J.P. MARVIN[1], C.F. KRECHTING[1], E.N. VAN LOO[1], A. LOMMEN[2], and O. DOLSTRA[1]
[1]*DLO-Centre for Plant Breeding and Reproduction Research (CPRO-DLO), P.O. Box 16, NL-6700 AA Wageningen, The Netherlands.*
[2]*State Institute for Quality Control of Agricultural Products (RIKILT-DLO). P.O. Box 230, NL-6700 AE Wageningen, The Netherlands.*

Summary

Reduction of ammonia emission from manure is an important issue in the Netherlands. Dairy husbandry is responsible for approximately 90% of the total ammonia emission in the Netherlands which is mainly due to poor utilization of nitrogen from the feed. Supplementation of forage maize to the ration of grazing cattle will increase the energy supply in the rumen and thereby increase the animal performance and decrease ammonia emission. Only 50–70% of the cell walls from maize stalks is degraded in the rumen. Factors limiting cell wall degradation are not yet fully understood. By studying fermentation characteristics of recombinant inbred lines of maize (RILs), we aim to get a better understanding of the factors in the cell wall determining its fermentation and their genetic control. Flour samples of the stalk fraction of 25 different RILs were incubated in rumen fluid *in vitro* after which the following fermentation characteristics were determined: organic matter digestibility (Dv%), cell wall digestibility (Dcw%), and composition and concentration of phenolic acids in the supernatant. The RILs varied greatly in Dv% (62–80%) and Dcw% (44–62%). The lignin content of the stalk-cell walls correlated negatively with both Dv% ($r = -0.79$) and Dcw% ($r = -0.66$) and positively with neutral detergent fiber content (NDF: $r = 0.66$). ^{1}H-NMR and HPLC analysis of the supernatant fluid after incubation of stalk-cell walls of RILs in an *in vitro* incubation with rumen fluid, revealed the presence of the following phenolic acids: phenylacetic acid, p-hydroxyphenylacetic acid, 3-phenylpropionic acid, 3-[4-hydroxyphenyl]propionic acid, p-coumaric acid, ferulic acid, p-hydroxybenzoic acid, vanillic acid, and syringic acid. A high correlation of phenylacetic acid and the branched volatile fatty acid, isobutyrate, suggests that this phenolic acid is derived from protein degradation. Isolation of phenolic acids from cell free rumen fluid was affected by an alkaline treatment of the supernatant fluid. It is suggested that cell free rumen fluid contains binding sites for phenolic acids which influence the extraction efficiency of phenolic acids from rumen fluid.

Ammonia emission from manure

In the last 20–30 years dairy husbandry in West-Europe has strongly been intensified. This intensification has led to negative effects on the environment due to increased production of manure. High losses of mineral nutrients into the environment occur from manure (e.g. ammonia). Emission of nitrogenoxides, sulfuroxides and ammonia causes acidification of surface water, resulting in dead lakes such as found in Scandinavia, disturbance of ecosystems in the soil and forest death. In addition, surplus of nitrate may lead to pollution of surface and soil water resources for drinking water.

Oudendag and Wijnands (31) reported that in the year 1980 about 240,000 tons ammonia was emitted into the air in the Netherlands. At present the emission is estimated to be approximately 200,000 tons. Animal manure is estimated to cause 90% of the Dutch ammonia emission (29). The impact of this alarming high ammonia emission made the Dutch government decide to intervene. The goals of ammonia emission reduction and the timespan which was set to reach these goals are set out in the Dutch national environmental policy plan NMP (National Milieubeleids Plan). In this plan the Dutch government aims for a reduction of the ammonia emission to 50–70% of the emission levels in 1980 by the year 2000 (3). The need to reduce nitrogen emission from manure has also been recognized by other European countries, but no formal regulations have been proposed to achieve a reduction (34). Only Belgium (Flanders) aims to reach a 60% reduction in the year 2010 compared to levels in 1980.

In the Netherlands cattle husbandry is responsible for about 60% of the total national ammonia emission (31) which is mainly due to the low efficiency of nitrogen uptake from the feed. Less than 20% of the nitrogen that enters the Dutch dairy farm is converted to milk and beef (1). The remainder is lost to the environment as ammonia volatilization, nitrate leaking, and denitrification. A better balance between the rate of protein degradation and the rate of release of energy from plant material in the rumen of cattle is needed to improve the utilisation of nitrogen from the feed by ruminants.

The average daily ration of ruminants in the Netherlands consists of approximately 50% grass, 10% forage maize and 40% concentrates (25). Nitrogen utilisation by ruminants when fed on grass only is rather poor, because of the relatively low energy content of grass. To improve nitrogen utilisation, the ration needs energy-rich supplements. Maize silage is very popular for this purpose because of its high energy and low protein content. Supplementation with maize silage in the ration of grazing cows can reduce the nitrogen excretion by 30–35% (39). The increasing popularity of maize silage to improve animal performance is clearly demonstrated by the explosive increase of its acreage in the last few decades. Since 1972 the acreage of maize grown in the Netherlands increased from 29,000 ha to about 230,000 ha in 1992 (4). The current cultivation results in a yearly forage production of about 3 million tons. Nearly half the production consists of cell walls with a ruminal degradability of about 50%. This implies a contribution to the national manure production of 3/4 million tons. Hence, improvements of the fodder quality of maize implies predominantly improvement of the ruminal digestion of cell walls. To accomplish this improvement, a better understanding of the factors limiting the cell wall digestion is essential. Once these factors are known, the genetics behind digestibility of cell walls can be identified and this knowledge can be used to alter and improve the fodder quality of maize.

Factors affecting ruminal cell wall digestibility

CELL WALL CONSTITUENTS

Cell walls of forages contain polysaccharides and aromatic compounds such as lignin and phenolic acids (16,17,19). Lignin content as well as the content of the major cell wall phenolic acids, p-coumaric and ferulic acid, have been shown to correlate negatively with forage digestibility (8,16,20). Within the cell wall, easily degradable structural carbohydrates are crosslinked to simple phenolic monomers (p-coumaric and ferulic acid) and core lignin (19). Crosslinking of lignin and carbohydrates by phenolic acids makes the cell wall more rigid and more resistant to microbial degradation (19). Although lignin and phenolic acids in the cell wall affect cell wall digestibility negatively, not all variation observed for cell wall digestibility can be explained by the amount of these constituents in the cell wall alone (24). The cell wall architecture may play a significant role as well. Nevertheless, it is expected that improvement of cell wall digestibility of forages may be realised by changing the amount and composition of lignin and phenolic acids in the cell wall.

PHENOLICS RELEASED FROM THE CELL WALL

During fermentation of forage cell walls, phenolic-carbohydrate complexes are released from the cell wall, both in vitro and in vivo (13, 18, 21, 22, 30). Perhaps the major cell wall phenolic acids, p-coumaric and ferulic acid are also released, but so far free p-coumaric and ferulic acid have been detected only in trace amounts in rumen fluid in vivo (21). Phenolic-carbohydrate complexes as well as free p-coumaric and ferulic acid have been shown to have a negative effect on digestion (2, 9, 18, 20, 37). In addition, several studies have also shown an inhibitory effect of carbohydrate esters of phenolic acids (5, 23, 33). Although the concentrations of free p-coumaric and ferulic acid observed are much lower than the concentrations needed to evoke inhibition of digestibility (9, 21, 22), it is believed that fibrolytic microorganisms, when attached to the cell wall, might be exposed to toxic levels of free phenolic acids (9). Non-specific absorption of free phenolic acids to microbial surfaces, and/or accumulation and fermentation of p-coumaric and ferulic acid into less toxic compounds by hydrogenation of the double bond in the propenoic side chain and subsequent breakdown to 3-phenylpropionic acid has been suggested to explain the low concentration of free p-coumaric and ferulic acid in the rumen (9).

INVOLVEMENT OF ANAEROBIC FUNGI IN CELL WALL DIGESTIBILITY

Rumen fluid contains a diversity of microorganisms which all contribute to the degradation of plant cell walls. Among these, the anaerobic fungi play a prominent role in degradation of lignin-rich cell walls because of the synergistic action of a wide range of hydrolysing enzymes produced by these organisms (40). Especially the recently discovered fungi esterases, p-coumaroyl and feruloyl esterases, may be important for the ability of the fungi to weaken and degrade extensively lignified tissue. These esterases cleave ferulic or p-coumaric acid from arabinoxylans (7) and are not or in very low amounts present in fiber degrading rumen bacteria (6). Although rumen fungi solubilize phenolic compounds from the cell wall, they cannot utilize these compounds for growth (14).

CPRO-DLO programme on maize fodder quality

CPRO-DLO is involved in a large multi-disciplinary programme on fodder quality of grass, which is carried out by several DLO institutes and the Agricultural University of Wageningen. DLO stands for Agricultural Research Service of the Ministry of Agriculture, Nature Management and Fisheries. The main objective of this programme is to decrease the ammonia emission from manure in the Netherlands. CPRO-DLO participates in this programme with studies on ruminal digestibility of maize and grasses. It is expected that the ammonia emission can be reduced significantly by genetic improvement of the degree of degradation of cell walls of maize and grasses. In order to do so, the genetics of differences in cell wall digestibility, chemical and physical characteristics of cell walls must be determined. To perform such studies with maize we have generated a series of recombinant inbred lines (RILs) by repeated selfing of the F_1 between the homozygous parent inbred lines Co125 (poorly digestible) and W401 (highly digestible) without any intentional selection. The resulting RILs are nearly homozygous due to this continuous process of selfing (11). The fermentation properties of 25 different RILs were determined in an *in vitro* assay with rumen fluid. Characteristics such as organic matter digestibility (Dv%), stalk-cell wall digestibility (Dcw%), volatile fatty acid (VFA) production and release of phenolic acids from the cell wall were recorded. The genetic aim of the RIL study is to detect and locate the genetic factors controlling the degradation of maize cell walls, amongst others using molecular markers such as RFLP's (restriction fragment length polymorphism). In addition, these lines will indicate which biochemical characteristics of cell walls in maize are likely to respond to breeding and selection.

The first results on the phenolic acid composition in the supernatants of RILs after digestion by rumen microorganisms *in vitro* as determined by HPLC and ^{1}H-NMR have been obtained and will be described.

Digestibility of recombinant inbred lines *in vitro*

EFFECT OF LIGNIN CONTENT

Ground material from the stalk fraction of 25 different RILs was incubated in triplo with rumen fluid for 48 hours according to the method of van Soest *et al.* (38), after which organic matter digestibility (Dv%) and cell wall digestibility (Dcw%) were determined.

The RILs varied greatly in organic matter digestibility (Dv%: 62–80%) and stalk-cell wall digestibility (Dcw%: 44–62%). It is known that lignin content of the cell wall correlates negatively with digestibility (19). To verify whether this is also true for the RILs of maize, the permanganate lignin content of the stalk-cell wall was determined. The lignin content of RILs ranged from 25 to 57 g/kg dry matter and was negatively correlated with both Dv% and Dcw% ($r= -0.79$ and -0.66, respectively; $p<0.01$) and positively with the neutral detergent fiber content (NDF: $r= 0.66$; $p<0.01$) (Fig. 3.1).

PHENOLIC ACID COMPOSITION IN SUPERNATANT FLUID AS DETERMINED BY ¹H-NMR

We have used ¹H-NMR to identify and quantify all soluble free phenolic acid monomers present in the supernatant fluid of RILs after

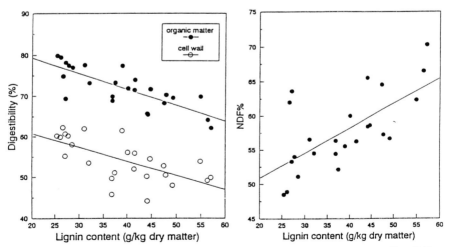

Figure 3.1. Correlation between lignin content and organic matter- and cell wall digestibility (Dv% and Dcw%, respectively) and cell wall content (NDF) from 25 different recombinant inbred lines (RILs) from maize.

digestion by rumen microorganisms *in vitro*. Phenylacetic acid, 3-phenylpropionic acid and p-hydroxyphenylacetic acid were the only phenolic acids which could be detected in the supernatant fluid by this method. Large differences between the RILs were observed for all three phenolic acids. The highest concentration was found for 3-phenylpropionic acid (0.57–1.41 mM), phenylacetic acid was present in concentrations of 0.32–0.46 mM and p-hydroxyphenylacetic acid in concentrations of 71–105 μM. Chesson *et al.* (9) observed the same phenolic acids in similar concentrations in rumen liquid from grass-fed sheep. In contrast to our observation with ¹H-NMR, Chesson *et al.* (9) also showed the presence of 3–[4-hydroxyphenyl]propionic acid which was suggested to be produced by hydrogenation of the double bond in the propenoic side chain of cinnamic acids (p-coumaric and ferulic acid). These hydrogenated products were found to be less toxic to rumen microorganisms than their putative parent compounds. A further modification of added cinnamic acids did not occur in the *in vitro* incubations (9).

Detoxification of cinnamic acids by hydrogenation, followed by dehydroxylation and demethoxylation to yield 3-phenylpropionic acid has been suggested to occur in the rumen (10, 26). This hypothesis was confirmed by later experiments of Martin (27) who observed an increase in concentration of 3-phenylpropionic acid in rumen fluid when cinnamic acids were infused into the rumen. 3-Phenylpropionic acid has been reported as the major phenolic acid in rumen fluid (32, 35) and appears to stimulate growth of some ruminal microorganisms (15, 36). A total transition to 3-phenylpropionic acid of all p-coumaric and ferulic acid which are released from cell walls of RILs after degradation in our *in vitro* incubation, could give rise to approximately 0.6–1.1 mM 3-phenylpropionic acid. This amount is close to the observed concentration for this phenolic acid (0.57–1.41 mM).

On the other hand, 3-phenylpropionic acid as well as phenylacetic acid and p-hydroxyphenylacetic acid have been postulated as fermentation products of protein degradation in the rumen (35). By means of a Stickland reaction the amino acids tyrosine and phenylalanine may be transited into phenylacetic acid, p-hydroxyphenylacetic acid and 3–[4-hydroxyphenyl]propionic acid in the rumen (35). We observed a strong correlation between the amount of phenylacetic acid and the branched fatty acid, isobutyrate ($r = 0.90$) in the supernatants of RILs. As protein degradation by rumen microorganism has been reported to yield branched volatile fatty acids such as isobutyrate (12) it is likely that the major part of the phenylacetic acid in the supernatants of

RILs is derived from protein degradation. 3-Phenylpropionic acid and p-hydroxyphenylacetic acid did not correlate well with isobutyrate ($r = 0.37$ and 0.1, respectively). These phenolic acids might have been formed from various sources, e.g. through protein degradation and partial degradation of cell wall phenolic acids. As ^{1}H-NMR, with the conditions used in our studies, only detects soluble phenolic acids in concentrations above roughly 10 μM, part of the phenolic acids in the supernatants of RILs will not be identified and quantified in this way. Phenolic acids below this detection limit and phenolic acids esterified to large carbohydrates or accumulated in and on rumen microbes will escape detection.

PHENOLIC ACID COMPOSITION IN SUPERNATANT FLUID AS DETERMINED BY HPLC

HPLC, in combination with extraction of phenolic acids from the supernatant fluid, will allow detection of much lower concentrations of soluble phenolic acids compared to ^{1}H-NMR. If the phenolic acid extraction is preceded by an alkaline hydrolysis, esterified and bound phenolic acids can be quantified as well. An HPLC analysis of an ether extract of a supernatant of a RIL after incubation with rumen fluid and after a subsequent alkaline treatment is shown in Fig. 3.2. By means of comparison with retention times of pure commercial compounds and by ^{1}H-NMR analysis of the ether extract, several peaks in the HPLC chromatogram could be identified. The following phenolic acids were identified: p-hydroxybenzoic acid, 3–[4-hydroxyphenyl]propionic acid, vanillic acid, syringic acid, p-hydroxyphenylacetic acid, p-coumaric acid, ferulic acid, phenylacetic acid and 3-phenylpropionic acid. The presence of vanillic and syringic acid in the liquid phase after fermentation of cell walls has been reported before (18). *p*-Coumaric and ferulic acids were not found when the alkaline treatment was omitted which suggests that these two phenolic acids were esterified to carbohydrate-lignin complexes or bound to proteins and/or microbe surfaces.

EFFECT OF AN ALKALINE HYDROLYSIS ON EXTRACTION RECOVERIES OF PHENOLIC ACIDS

It was observed that when the phenolic acid extraction was carried out without the alkaline pretreatment of the supernatant fluid, the recovery

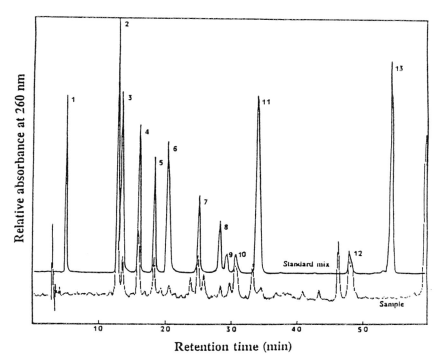

Figure 3.2. HPLC chromatograms of phenolic acids extracted from cell free rumen fluid of a RIL after a 48 hours incubation and a standard mix containing the following phenolic acids: gallic acid (1), p-hydroxybenzoic acid (2), p-hydroxyphenylacetic acid (3), vanillic acid (4), syringic acid (5), 3–[4-hydroxyphenyl]propionic acid (6), p-coumaric acid (7), ferulic acid (8), sinapic acid (9), phenylacetic acid (10), benzoic acid (11), 3-phenylpropionic acid (12) and trans-cinnamic acid (13).

of added phenolic acids by extraction decreased with decreasing amounts of added phenolic acids. This effect was most pronounced for p-coumaric acid and is shown in Table 3.1. Although to a smaller extent, this effect was also seen for other phenolic acids (not shown). The recovery remained high for the whole range, 0.4–6.7 µg/ml supernatant, when an alkaline treatment was included in the extraction procedure.

Ether alone can apparently not liberate all of these immobilized phenolic acids from their binding sites. Instead, a total destruction of the binding sites by hydrolysis with alkali is needed to allow accurate extraction and quantification. Complex formation of simple phenolics with enzymes/proteins by hydrophobic interactions, analogous to the complexes formed between tannin and proteins, has been postulated by McManus *et al.* (28). Perhaps proteins in the rumen which are coated

Table 3.1 RECOVERY OF P-COUMARIC ACID ADDED TO CELL FREE RUMEN FLUID WITH TWO DIFFERENT EXTRACTION PROCEDURES.

	Extraction procedure	
	No alkaline treatment p-Coumaric acid (% recovered)	Alkaline treatment p-Coumaric acid (% recovered)
Amount (μg)		
100	79	82
75	79	86
50	76	88
25	74	88
12.5	58	92
6.3	52	100

p-Coumaric acid was added to 15 ml cell free rumen fluid.

with simple phenolic acids might escape ruminal degradation. This could result in improved utilization of the feed nitrogen by the ruminants. Thus, phenolic acids in rumen fluid might influence ruminal digestion of plant material but they might also improve nitrogen utilization by ruminants from their feed by protecting proteins from ruminal degradation resulting in decreased ammonia emission and improved animal performance.

Future research

Correlation studies in this report show that lignin content of the cell wall of RILs can explain 62 and 44% of the variation in Dv% and Dcw%, respectively. In the near future we plan to study the contribution of cell wall phenolic acids to the observed variation in Dv% and Dcw%.

In addition we concluded that proteins which are added to the rumen fluid in the *in vitro* assay according to van Soest as nitrogen source are partially fermented to phenolic acids. This phenomenon may influence the fermentation process of the cell walls of RILs. Therefore, the same studies will be performed with supplementation of ammonia as nitrogen source instead of proteins.

To obtain data on heritability of fermentation characteristics of RILs, *in vitro* incubations will be repeated with the same set of RILs grown in another trial. Further studies will also aim to separate the role of bacteria and fungi in digestion of plant cell wall material.

References

(1) AARTS, H.F.M., BIEWINGA, E.D., BRUIN, G., EDEL, B. and KOREVAAR, H. (1988). Melkveehouderij en milieu. Rapport 111, Proefstation voor de Rundveehouderij, Schapenhouderij en Paardenhouderij, Lelystad, The Netherlands.

(2) AKIN, D.E. (1982). Forage cell wall degradation and p-coumaric, ferulic and sinapic acids. Agronomy Journal 74, 424–428.

(3) ANONYMOUS. (1989). Nationaal Milieubeleidsplan. Tweede Kamer vergaderjaar 198801989, 21 137, nrs.1–2 p. 134, SDU Uitgeverij, Den Haag, The Netherlands.

(4) ANONYMOUS. (1993). 67e Beschrijvende Rassenlijst voor Landbouwgewassen 1993. Leiter-Nijpels b.v., Maastricht, The Netherlands.

(5) BOHN, P.J. and FALES, S.L. (1989). Cinnamic acid-carbohydrate esters: an evaluation of a model system. Journal of the Science of Food and Agriculture 48, 1–7.

(6) BORNEMAN, W.S. and AKIN, D.E. (1990). Lignocellulose degradation by rumen fungi and bacteria, pp. 325–339. In (D.E. Akin *et al.*,ed.): Microbial and plant opportunities to improve lignocellulose utilization by ruminants, Elsevier Sci. Publ. Co., New York.

(7) BORNEMAN, W.S., LJUNGDAHL, L.G., HARTLEY, R.D. and AKIN, D.E. (1991). Isolation and characterization of p-coumaroyl esterase from the anaerobic fungus *Neocallimastix* strain MC-2. Applied and Environmental Microbiology 57, 2337–2344.

(8) BURRITT, E.A., BITTNER, A.S, STREET, J.C. and ANDERSON, M.J. (1984). Correlations of phenolic acids and xylose content of cell wall with in vitro dry matter digestibility of three maturing grasses. Journal of Dairy Science 67, 1209–1213.

(9) CHESSON, A., STEWART, C.S. and WALLACE R.J. (1982). Influence of plant phenolic acids on growth and cellulolytic activity of rumen bacteria. Applied and Environmental Microbiology 44, 597–603.

(10) CHESTNUT, A.B., FAHEY, G.C.Jr., BERGER, L.L. and SPEARS, J.W. (1986). Effects of sulfur fertilization on composition and digestion of phenolic compounds in tall fescue and orchardgrass. Journal of Animal Science 63, 1926–1934.

(11) DOLSTRA, O., VAN DER PUTTEN, P.E.L. and MEDEMA, J.H. (1991). Genetics of cell wall digestibility in forage maize.

pA23. In: Abstracts of international symposium on forage cell wall structure and digestibility. 7–10 oct. Madison WI, US. Dairy Forage Research Center Madison, WI, USA.

(12)   EL-SHAZLY, K. (1952). Degradation of protein in the rumen of sheep. 2. The action of rumen micro-organisms on amino-acids. Biochemical Journal 51, 647–653.

(13)   GAILLARD, B.D.E. and RICHARDS, G.N. (1975). Presence of soluble lignin-carbohydrate complexes in the bovine rumen. Carbohydrate Research 42, 135–145.

(14)   GORDON, G.L.R. and PHILLIPS, M.W. (1989). Degradation and utilization of cellulose and straw by three different anaerobic fungi from the ovine rumen. Applied and Environmental Microbiology 55, 1703–1710.

(15)   GOROSITO, A.R., RUSSELL, J.B. and VAN SOEST, P.J. (1985). Effect of carbon-4 and carbon-5 volatile fatty acids on digestion of plant cell wall in vitro. Journal of Dairy Science 68, 840–847.

(16)   HARTLEY, R.D. (1972). p-Coumaric and ferulic acid components of cell walls of ryegrass and their relatioships with lignin and digestibility. Journal of the Science of Food and Agriculture 23, 1347–1354.

(17)   HARTLEY, R.D. (1981). Chemical constitution, properties and processing of lignocellulose wastes in relation to nutritional quality for animals. Agriculture and Environment 6, 91–113.

(18)   JUNG, H-.G. (1988). Inhibitory potential of phenolic-carbohydrate complexes released during ruminal fermentation. Journal of Agricultural and Food Chemistry 36, 782–788.

(19)   JUNG, H-.G. (1989). Forage lignins and their effects on fiber digestibility. Agronomy Journal 81, 33–38.

(20)   JUNG, H-.G. and FAHEY, G.C. Jr. (1983). Interactions among phenolic monomers and in vitro fermentation. Journal of Dairy Science 66, 1255–1263.

(21)   JUNG, H-.G., FAHEY, G.C. JR. and GARST, J.E. (1983). Simple phenolic monomers of forages and effects of in vitro fermentation on cell wall phenolics. Journal of Animal Science 57, 1294–1305.

(22)   JUNG, H-.G., FAHEY, G.C.JR., and MERCHEN, N.R. (1983). Effects of ruminant digestion and metabolism on phenolic monomers of forages. British Journal of Nutrition 50, 637–651.

(23)   JUNG, H-.G. and SAHLU, T. (1986). Depression of cellulose

digestion by esterified cinnamic acids. Journal of the Science of Food and Agriculture 37, 659–665.

(24)   JUNG, H-.G. and RUSSELLE, M.P. (1991). Light source and nutrient regime effects on fiber composition and digestibility of forages. Crop Science 31, 1065–1070.

(25)   KETELAARS, J.J.M.H. and VAN VUUREN, A.M. (1989). Hoge prioriteit voor onderzoek naar graskwaliteit. Meststoffen 2/3, 21–30.

(26)   MARTIN, A.K., MILNE, J.A. and MOBERLEY, P. (1975). Urinary quinol and orcinol output as indices of voluntary intake of heather (*Calluna vulgaris* L. (Hull)) by sheep. Proceedings of Nutrition Society 34, 70A-71A.

(27)   MARTIN, A.K. (1982). The origin of urinary aromatic compounds excreted by ruminants. 1. The metabolism of quinic, cyclohexanecarboxylic and non-phenolic aromatic acids to benzoic acid. British Journal of Nutrition 47, 139–154.

(28)   MCMANUS, J.P., DAVIS, K.G., LILLEY, T.H. and HASLAM, E. (1981). The association of proteins with polyphenols. Journal of the Chemical Society Chemical Communications pp. 309.

(29)   MILIEUVERKENNING. (1988). Zorgen voor morgen: nationale milieuverkenning 1985–2010. F. Langeweg (ed.). Samson H.D., Tjeenk Willink, Alphen aan de Rijn, The Netherlands.

(30)   NEILSON, M.J. and RICHARDS, G.N. (1978). The fate of the soluble lignin-carbohydrate complex produced in the bovine rumen. Journal of the Science of Food and Agriculture 29, 513–519.

(31)   OUDENDAG, D.A. and WIJNANDS, J.H.M. (1989). Beperking van de ammoniakemissie uit dierlijk mest: een verkenning van de mogelijkheden en kosten. LEI-DLO, onderzoekverslag 56, Den Haag, The Netherlands.

(32)   PATTON, S. and KESLER E.M. (1967). Presence and significance of phenyl-substituted fatty acids in bovine rumen contents. Journal of Dairy Science 50, 1505–1508.

(33)   SAWAI, A., KONDO, T. and ARA, S. (1983). Inhibitory effects of phenolic acid esters on degradability of forage fibers. Journal of Japanese Society for Grassland Science 29, 175–179.

(34)   SCHRÖDER, J. (1992). Legislation on animal manure in Europe. Meststoffen, 69–74.

(35)   SCOTT, T.W., WARD, P.F.V. and DAWSON, R.M.C. (1964).

The formation and metabolism of phenyl-substituted fatty acids in the rumen. Biochemical Journal 90, 12–24.

(36)   STACK, R.J. and COTTA, M.A. (1986). Effect of 3-phenyl-propionic acid on growth of and cellulose utilization by cellulolytic ruminal bacteria. Applied and Environmental Microbiology 52, 209–210.

(37)   THEODOROU, M.K., GASCOYNE, D.J., AKIN, D.E. and HARTLEY, R.D. (1987). Effect of phenolic acids and phenolics from plant cell walls on rumen-like fermentation in consecutive batch culture. Applied and Environmental Microbiology 53, 1046–1050.

(38)   VAN SOEST, P.J., WINE R.H. and MOORE L.A. (1966). Estimation of true digestibility of forages by the in vitro digestion of cell walls, pp. 438–441. In: Proc. 10th Int. Grassland Congress, Helsinki.

(39)   VAN VUUREN, A.M. and MEIJS, J.A.C. (1987). Effects of herbage composition and supplement feeding on the excretion of nitrogen in dung and urine by grazing dairy cows, pp. 17–24. In (H.G. van der Meer, R.J. Unwin, T.A. van Dijk and G.C. Ennik, eds.): Animal manure on grassland and fodder crops, Martinus Nijhoff Publishers, Dordrecht, The Netherlands.

(40)   WUBAH, D.A., AKIN, D.E. and BORNEMAN, W.S. (1993). Biology, fiber-degradation, and enzymology of anaerobic zoosporic fungi. Critical Reviews in Microbiology 19, 99–115.

4

MICROBIAL AND CHEMICAL CHARACTERIZATION OF RUMEN CONTENTS OF GRAZING DAIRY COWS

F. MARTILLOTTI, S. TERRAMOCCIA, C. TRIPALDI, S. PUPPO
and V. DANESE
Istituto Sperimentale per la Zootecnia, Rome, Italy

Summary

Rumen fluid from three fistulated grazing Friesian dairy cows was sampled in different seasons (autumn, late spring, early summer), to determine VFA, NH_3, pH, buffer capacity (BC) and the total numbers of bacteria and fungi. Forage samples were incubated in nylon bags in the rumen for 0, 1, 2, 4, 8, 16, 24, 48, 72 h to determine the crude protein and NDF degradability kinetics. The values of the VFA and NH_3 contents diminished from 8.00 to 16.00 h (11.16 vs 7.5 mmol%; 1.48 vs 1.22 mmol% respectively). The total bacteria numbers were significantly higher in the autumn than in the other seasons. The total number of fungi was significantly higher in the autumn than in the other seasons only in samples obtained at 08.00 h; in the spring, the total number of fungi was higher at 20.00 than at other times.

Introduction

The energetic efficiency of microbial growth was at one time thought to be constant, but is now accepted as variable depending both on microbial species and growth condition in the rumen. The attention of nutritionists is therefore focused on chemical and physical rumen parameters to better explain how they affect microbial growth (7, 9).

Until now, studies on ruminal parameters in grazing animals are few, especially in Italy where seasonal climatic variations, including long dry periods, cause drastic changes in the feeding value of pastures.

This study represents the beginning of more complete research having as its main purpose determining energy and protein supplemental demands of extensively-fed ruminants in different climatic conditions.

Materials and methods

The trial was carried out with three dry fistulated friesian dairy cows, grazing on permanent meadow, in three different seasons: autumn, late spring and early summer.

Volatile fatty acids were determined by HPLC after filtration with 0.45 μm membrane filters (4). Ammonia was determined after steam distillation on Mg0 (5). pH and buffer capacity (BC) were determined according to (3) and expressed as mequiv. H^+%). Total bacterial numbers were determined anaerobically on Petri dishes using the complete medium of Leedle (2); fungi were enumerated using the Joblin roll bottle method (1).

The rates of crude protein and neutral detergent fibre (NDF) degradation were determined on forage collected from the same pasture, chopped, weighed in nylon bags (30 g/10 × 13 cm) and incubated in the rumen for 0, 1, 2, 4, 8, 16, 24, 48, 72 hours.

The kinetics of crude protein (CP) and NDF degradability were computed using the Ørskov and Macdonald (8) equation and by the logarithmic linearization procedure of Nocek and English (6).

The experimental design was:

$$Yijk = M + Ai + Bj + (AB)ij + Eijk \text{ where:}$$

A = seasons (i = 1 .... 3); B = sampling times (j = 1 .... 6); for bacterial and fungal numbers B = sampling times (j = 1 .... 3); M = mean; k = no. of observations; E = error)

Results

The concentrations of VFA and NH_3 in the rumen of the animals studied were affected both by the season, and by the time of sampling. For the VFA, during springtime the highest concentrations were found at 04:00 and 08:00h: these were the highest concentrations of VFA recorded throughout the seasons studied. In the summer, the peak concentration of VFA was found at 24:00h. In the autumn, the highest

Table 4.1 CHEMICAL PARAMETERS (%) IN RUMEN FLUID SAMPLED EVERY 4 HOURS IN DIFFERENT SEASONS

	8:00	12:00	16:00	20:00	24:00	04:00
VFA (mM)						
Aut.	$^a10.13_a$	$^a9.11_a$	$^a9.47_a$	$^a8.38_a$	$^a6.62_a$	$^b6.02_a$
Spr.	$^a13.28_{ab}$	$^a7.48_{bc}$	$^a6.48_c$	$^a8.97_{bc}$	$^a7.27_{bc}$	$^a14.10_a$
Sum.	$^a10.07_a$	$^a7.52_{ab}$	$^a6.18_b$	$^a6.56_b$	$^a12.17_a$	$^b8.70_{ab}$
NH₃(mM)						
Aut.	$^a2.33_a$	$^a2.13_a$	$^a2.19_a$	$^a1.45_b$	$^a1.20_b$	$^a1.00_b$
Spr.	$^b1.59_a$	$^b1.41_{ab}$	$^b0.95_{bc}$	$^a1.03_{abc}$	$^b0.51_c$	$^a1.13_{ab}$
Sum.	$^c0.53_a$	$^c0.43_a$	$^b0.51_a$	$^b0.35_a$	$^b0.19_a$	$^b0.35_a$
pH						
Aut.	$^b6.66_{bc}$	$^b6.60_{bc}$	$^b6.39_c$	$^b6.77_{abc}$	$^a7.05_{ab}$	$^a7.23_a$
Spr.	$^{ab}6.96_a$	$^a7.38_a$	$^{ab}7.40_a$	$^{ab}7.21_a$	$^a7.33_a$	$^a6.92_a$
Sum.	$^a7.26_a$	$^a7.40_a$	$^a7.66_a$	$^a7.39_a$	$^a7.33_a$	$^a7.39_a$
BC (meq H⁺)						
Aut.	$^a12.08_a$	$^a12.70_a$	$^a13.26_a$	$^a12.49_a$	$^a12.13_a$	$^{ab}12.04_a$
Spr.	$^a14.14_a$	$^a12.79_{ab}$	$^a12.21_{ab}$	$^a12.79_{ab}$	$^{ab}11.94_a$	$^a13.83_{ab}$
Sum.	$^a12.25_a$	$^b10.21_{bc}$	$^b9.30_c$	$^b9.61_{bc}$	$^b10.12_{bc}$	$^b11.36_{ab}$

a, b, c: P = 0.05 superscripts refer to the seasons (columns), subscripts refer to the sampling times (rows)

concentration of VFA was found at 08:00h, and the lowest concentration was found at 04:00 h. The most striking differences between the seasons was therefore the differences in the pattern of diurnal fluctuation of the VFA concentrations, and the trend for the values in springtime to be slightly (but not always significantly) higher than at other times of the year. The amounts of ammonia were greater in autumn than in spring, and for much of the day (Table 4.1) greater in spring than in summer. The concentrations of ammonia found were highest at 08:00 in all of the seasons studied. The seasonal differences in VFA and NH_3 concentrations in the rumen presumably reflect the state of the pasture herbage, which would have been comparatively young and highly digestible in the spring, but of lower degradability in the summer and autumn.

The rumen pH was affected by the season, and tended to be higher in the summer than at other times of year. The buffer capacity of the rumen contents tended to be lower when the rumen pH was high and vice versa. The study of crude protein (CP) and NDF degradability (Table 4.2) showed values that decreased from autumn-spring-summer (76.30, 65.68 and 25.95% for CP and 61.68, 43.25 and 24.77% for NDF respectively) according to the vegetative phase of the samples of pasture herbage used. The total numbers of viable bacteria and fungi in the rumen tended to be higher in autumn than in spring or summer (Table 4.3). The peak population sizes thus tended to occur when the

Table 4.2   KINETICS AND STATISTICAL DATA OF PROTEIN AND NDF RUMEN DEGRADABILITY

	a	b	c	l	r^2	RSD	P%
CP							
Aut.	42.16	52.11	0.095	–	0.97	4.43	76.30
Spr.	16.33	75.33	0.095	–	0.98	5.06	65.68
Sum.	19.90	11.17	0.150	6.5	0.95	1.20	25.95
NDF							
Aut.	21.48	63.85	0.085	–	0.98	3.99	61.68
Spr.	7.53	60.87	0.071	–	0.98	3.50	43.25
Sum.	2.80	49.44	0.040	–	0.98	2.67	24.77

P = observed degradability; a = zero time intercept (may approximate to soluble matter); b = potential degradability at infinite time minus a; c= degradation rate constant of b; l = lag (h); r = correlation coefficient; RSD = residual standard deviation.

Table 4.3   TOTAL BACTERIA ($\times 10^8$) AND FUNGAL ($\times 10^5$) NUMBERS IN WHOLE RUMEN CONTENT

	8:00	14:00	20:00
Bacteria			
Aut.	[a]333.33_a	[a]165.00_b	[a]359.67_a
Spr.	[b]24.25_a	[b]20.04_a	[b]21.67_a
Sum.	[b]0.74_a	[b]4.62_a	15.03_a
Fungi			
Aut.	[a]4.50_a	[a]0.55_b	[b]0.42_b
Spr.	[b]1.57_b	[a]1.78_a	[a]3.81_a
Sum.	[b]0.81_a	[a]0.65_a	[ab]1.90_a

a, b, c: P = 0.05 superscripts refer to the seasons (columns) and subscripts refer to the sampling times (rows)

concentrations of VFA and NH_3 in the rumen were high, and when the forage was being extensively degraded.

Conclusions

The differences between rumen NH_3 content, recorded among the three seasons, were much higher than the diurnal variations presumably because of the relatively small amounts of N in samples of late spring and summer forage.

The variation of VFA content among the period was much lower than that of NH_3 content, and the NH_3 content more than VFA content, affected pH and BC.

The CP and NDF effective degradability was different in the three periods and the highest c value was found with the summer forage for the crude protein and with the autumn forage for NDF.

The highest numbers of bacteria and fungi were recorded when NH_3 and VFA were present at high concentrations in the rumen.

This research was supported by NRC (Italy) Spec. Proj. RAISA, subproj. no. 3; paper no. 1007.

References

(1)   JOBLIN, K.M. (1981). Isolation enumeration and maintenance of rumen anaerobic fungi in roll tubes. Appl. Environ. Microbiol. 42, 1119–1122.

(2)   LEEDLE, J.A.Z., BRYANT, M.P. and HESPELL, R.B. (1982). Diurnal variations in bacterial numbers and fluid parameters in ruminal contents of animal fed low or high forage. Appl. Environ. Microbiol., 44, 402–412.

(3)   LE RUYET, P., TUCKER, W.B., HOGUE, J.F., ASLAM, M., LEMA, M., SHIN, I.S., MILLER, T.P. and ADAMS, G.D. (1992). Influence of dietary fiber and buffer value index on the ruminal milieu of lactating diary cows. J. Dairy Sci. 75, 2394–2407.

(4)   MARTILLOTTI, F. and PUPPO, S. (1985). Determinazione degli acidi organici negli insilati e nel rumine mediante cromatografia liquida ad alta risoluzione (HPLC). Ann. Inst. Sper. Zootech. 18, 1–10.

(5)   MARTILLOTTI, F., ANTONGIOVANNI, M., RIZZI, I., SANTI, E. and BITTANTE, G. (1987). Metodi di analisi per la valutazione degli alimenti di interesse zootecnico. Quaderni Metodologici no. 8. CNR-IPRA. Roma.

(6)   NOCEK, J.E. and ENGLISH, J.E. (1986). *In situ* degradation kinetics: evaluation of rate determination procedure. J. Dairy Sci. 69, 77–87.

(7)   OLDHAM, J.D. (1984). Protein-energy interelationships in dairy cows. J. Dairy Sci. 67, 1090–1114.

(8)   ØRSKOV, E.R. and MCDONALD, I. (1978). The estimation of protein degradability in rumen from incubation measurements weighted according to rate of passage. J. Agric. Sci. (Camb.) 92, 499–503.

(9)   VAN VUUREN, A.M. (1990). Nutrient supply from fresh herbage to dairy cows. Annual report by Agric. Res. Dep. Research Institute for An. Nutr. and Res. (IVVO-DLO).

5

DEGRADATION OF PLANT CELL WALL POLYSACCHARIDES BY RUMEN BACTERIA

H.J. FLINT
Rowett Research Institute, Greenburn Road, Bucksburn, Aberdeen AB2 9SB, UK

Summary

Only a few species of ruminal bacteria are capable of degrading the cellulose and hemicellulose present in plant cell walls. We still understand relatively little about the enzyme systems that give these bacteria their fibre-degrading abilities, but detailed genetic and biochemical investigations indicate that these organisms carry multiple genes specifying polysaccharidase activities. While polysaccharidases from rumen bacteria are generally found to be related in sequence to those of other microbes, certain hemicellulases show an organisation of catalytic domains into multifunctional polypeptides that is found in few other organisms. It is also becoming apparent from molecular studies that a high degree of genetic divergence exists between many strains of the same rumen species. This is observed both with polysaccharidase gene sequences and, in some cases, with 16SrRNA sequences, and suggests that we should be cautious at this stage in extrapolating from a small number of strains and isolated genes.

Introduction

Anaerobic bacteria are acknowledged to play vital roles in the degradation of plant cell wall material in the rumen. In order to understand these roles it is necessary to consider the influence of plant anatomy and composition on the colonisation of substrates by the rumen microflora as well as the activities, ecology and population dynamics of the bacteria themselves. Not surprisingly, extrapolating from work *in vitro*

49

with pure bacterial cultures and simplified, purified substrates to the complex rumen ecosystem has proved a difficult step (12). At a molecular level the problem is to extrapolate from the study of single genes and gene products to activities of whole cells, and this in turn is proving an equally large challenge. This article will first consider briefly some of the complexities of fibre degradation by rumen bacteria before moving on to molecular aspects.

The substrates

The major structural polysaccharides of the plant cell wall only become available as sources of energy to the host animal through the activities of the rumen microflora. Figure 5.1 shows some of the enzyme activities known to be involved in the degradation of the most abundant structural polysaccharides. The chemical and physical characteristics of cell walls that determine their degradability vary between plant species and cultivars and can also differ radically between different stages of growth, anatomical fractions and cell types (8). Most cell

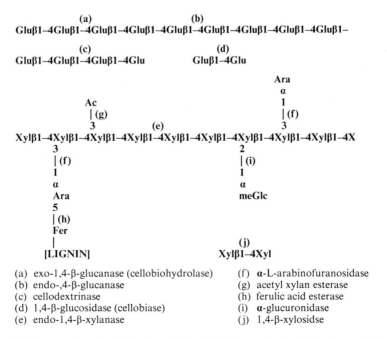

(a) exo-1,4-β-glucanase (cellobiohydrolase)   (f) α-L-arabinofuranosidase
(b) endo-,4-β-glucanase   (g) acetyl xylan esterase
(c) cellodextrinase   (h) ferulic acid esterase
(d) 1,4-β-glucosidase (cellobiase)   (i) α-glucuronidase
(e) endo-1,4-β-xylanase   (j) 1,4-β-xylosidse

Figure 5.1. Enzymes involved in the degradation of cellulose and xylan. [Glu glucose; Xyl xylose; Ara arabinofuranose; Ac acetyl group; Fer ferulic acid; meGlc 4-O-methyl glucuronic acid].

walls consist of cellulose fibrils embedded in a matrix of other poly-saccharides (hemicellulose and pectin) with varying amounts of lignification. The major matrix polysaccharides in particular vary widely in composition and structure. Xylan chains, for example, are substituted to varying degrees with arabinose, 4-O-methyl glucuronic acid and acetyl groupings. Thus a single 'enzyme activity', such as an endoxylanase, may cover a very wide range of enzymes varying in specificity and response to substituents on the main xylan chain (58) and activities involved in cleaving substituents play an important role in degradation. Different polysaccharides are interconnected within the cell wall via hydrogen bonding or glycosidic linkages, and connections to lignin may occur through phenolic acids linked via ester bonds to arabinose (28). In addition to cellulose, xylans and pectins, hem-icelluloses such as xyloglucans, arabinans and mixed linkage $\beta(1,3-1,4)$ glucans may be present together with protein and inorganic material.

Susceptibility of cell walls to microbial attack may be determined more by anatomical and physical features of the substrate, which influence the ability of cells to adhere and the accessibility of cell wall polysaccharides to degradative enzymes, than by fine variations in chemical structure (8). Bacterial degradation must be largely a super-ficial, erosive phenomenon since there is no evidence that cells and enzymes can penetrate the cell wall. A layer of material that may be only a minor component of the biomass can therefore play a very significant role in presenting a barrier to degradation.

The bacteria

DEGRADATION OF FORAGE CELL WALLS BY DIFFERENT SPECIES OF RUMEN BACTERIA

This topic has been recently reviewed (7, 12). Although the variability of substrates, and interstrain variation, complicate comparisons between species, certain generalisations can be made. Only three bacterial species commonly found in the rumen, *Fibrobacter succinogenes*, *Ruminococcus flavefaciens* and *Ruminococcus albus*, are generally to be considered cellulolytic, although other cellulolytic species have been reported. Many strains of these species cause extensive solubilisation of cellulose and hemicellulose from a wide range of forage material. *F. succinogenes* appears to form the closest association with cellulose fibrils (6). In addition some strains of two of the most numerous

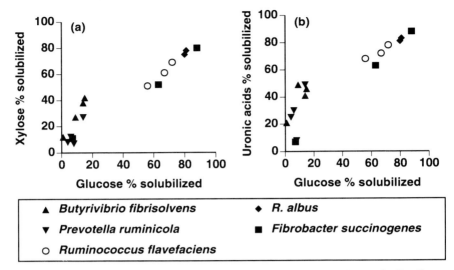

Figure 5.2. Solubilization of xylose (from hemicellulose) and uronic acids from teff cell walls as a function of glucose solubilization by pure cultures of rumen bacteria. [From data of Morris and van Gylswyk (43)]

bacterial species in the rumen, *Prevotella ruminicola* and *Butyrivibrio fibrisolvens*, although non-cellulolytic, are capable of solubilising a fraction of the hemicellulose and pectin present in some forages (12). In general, however, cellulolytic strains solubilise hemicellulose and pectin from forages to a greater degree than do non-cellulolytic strains (43) (Fig 5.2).

Relative numbers of cellulolytic bacteria are difficult to estimate reliably *in vivo* for a variety of reasons (52). *Ruminococci*, particularly *R. albus*, are almost invariably reported from animals fed fibrous rations, but *F. succinogenes* numbers may tend to be underestimated (54). The advent of molecular probing approaches based on 16SrRNA sequences promises to provide more convenient methods of enumeration in the long term (5, 16).

Synergistic interactions have been reported between different fibre degrading bacteria *in vitro* (11, 12). Whereas synergy with respect to utilisation of the breakdown products of pectin and hemicellulose can be quite dramatic, it is generally rather low at the level of degradation. If digestion occurs *in vivo* largely in the immediate vicinity of bacterial cells or homogenous microcolonies, as a function of cell bound enzyme complexes, then opportunities for the combined action of enzymes produced by different microbes may be limited. Synergistic effects may, however, result *in vivo* from a form of succession, in which initial colonisation by one organism 'unmasks' a substrate utilisable by a second organism (12) or as a consequence of cross-feeding of degradation products or metabolic end products. Negative interactions could be as important, or more important, *in vivo* (Stewart, this volume).

STRAIN VARIATION

It is important to stress that several rumen bacterial 'species' are known to conceal an enormous degree of interstrain genetic diversity. This is certainly true of *Prevotella ruminicola* and *Butyrivibrio fibrisolvens* which may each eventually need dividing into 9 or more new species (39, 41). We have found that certain *P. ruminicola* strains diverge in their 16SrRNA sequences to a greater degree than is typically found between different genera of Gram positive bacteria (3a). Clearly investigations based on single strains of each species cannot be relied upon to predict the behaviour of the majority of ruminal strains. Fortunately the phylogeny of *F. succinogenes* has now been put on a firm basis through molecular taxonomy (2, 51) although there are no such studies reported with ruminococci.

Most interstrain variation is assumed to reflect variation present in nature. However it is also clear that mutations can arise in laboratory cultures leading to significant activity changes (53). This suggests that adaptive changes occur continually both in the rumen and also during laboratory culture.

Genes and enzymes

ENZYME ACTIVITIES CONTRIBUTING TO PLANT CELL WALL DEGRADATION BY RUMEN BACTERIA

Despite the high activity of *F. succinogenes* cells against crystalline cellulose, cell free extracts show almost no activity, suggesting that some essential function or organisational feature is lost rapidly from non-growing cells. A range of cellulase components have been purified from strain S85 including two endoglucanases, a cellobiohydrolase/cellobiosidase and a cellodextrinase (20). The latter enzyme is periplasmic and appears to function in the utilisation of cello-oligosaccharides entering the cell.

R. flavefaciens cell extracts, or culture supernatants, retain rather more activity against crystalline cellulose (27). An exoglucanase (a dimer, subunit MW 118000) has been purified from *R. flavefaciens* FD1 that shows activity against insoluble cellulose (21). This strain produces multiple endoglucanases with as many as 18 different components estimated to be present in two separable complexes (13). There is evidence that some *R. flavefaciens* proteins are glycosylated, but it is not known if this applies to the degradative enzymes themselves (14). Endoglucanase activity was predominant in the extractable cellulase complex of *R. albus* SY3 (60) although a cellobiosidase showing exoglucanase action on soluble substrates has been purified from another *R. albus* strain (45).

Xylanase and pectinase activity is reported from all three cellulolytic species and from non-cellulolytic species such as *P. ruminicola* and *B. fibrisolvens*. Acetyl xylan esterase and phenolic acid esterase activities have been demonstrated in *F. succinogenes* (37) and acetyl xylan esterase in *B. fibrisolvens* (29); phenolic acid esterases were not found in *R. flavefaciens* FD1 (1).

CELLULOLYTIC BACTERIA AND CELLULOSOME ORGANISATION

Cellulolytic bacteria commonly carry high molecular weight surface structures, cellulosomes, which are visible by electron microscopy and which comprise many different polypeptides (34). These structures have only been studied in any detail in the non-rumen anaerobe *Clostridium thermocellum*. The cellulosome of *C. thermocellum* JW20 comprises as many as 26 different polypeptides ranging in apparent molecular weight from 37 to 190 kDa, 14 of which are glysosylated, and includes polypeptides having xylanase activity, others having endoglucanase activity and some having both activities (32). Polypeptides present within the cellulosome appear to carry a 23/24 amino acid sequence, repeated twice, which is thought to anchor them to a large 'scaffolding' protein (210 kDa) which in turn carries a cellulose binding domain. A cellobiohydrolase has also been reported from *C. thermocellum* (42). It still seems unclear, however, whether the ordered arrangement of different endoglucanase and binding components within the complex (9) is sufficient to explain the ability to degrade crystalline cellulose, or whether exoglucanase activity is an essential ingredient.

Synergy between exoglucanase (cellobiohydrolase) and endoglucanase components is known to be an essential feature of aerobic fungal cellulase systems (59).

The enzyme systems of the major cellulolytic rumen bacteria also appear to be present largely as high molecular weight aggregates (20, 47, 60) and cellulosome-like structures have been reported from *Ruminococcus albus* (34). There is a suggestion that *Butyrivibrio fibrisolvens* carries two distinct enzyme complexes on its cell surface, one of which has mainly xylanase and the other mainly endoglucanase activities (35).

One intriguing question raised by the cellulosome concept is how to account for the regulation of individual activities that occurs in response to growth on different substrates. In *R. albus* there is evidence that certain polypeptides are expressed preferentially on a given substrate (25) and xylanases are induced relative to CMCases in *R. flavefaciens* grown on xylan-containing substrates (18). Perhaps such inductions are due to enzymes not present within the cellulosome, or alternatively many different types of cellulosome structure may be formed depending on the chemical composition of the substrate.

ENZYME FAMILIES

The catalytic regions of polysaccharidase enzymes from a variety of microorganisms show similarities in their amino acid sequences and secondary structures that allow classification into enzyme families (24). Most actively cellulolytic organisms have generally been found to produce cellulase enzymes belonging to several different families (e.g. four in *C. thermocellum*). Furthermore enzymes from cellulolytic fungi and bacteria, or bacteria and plants, are in many cases found to belong within the same groups, suggesting that horizontal gene transfer may have played a role in their evolution. While catalytic domains and non-catalytic, cellulose-binding, domains show recognisable sequence conservation between species, other sequence elements are often found in the same polypeptide that are unique to a particular species (24). Some of these may be concerned, for example, with protein-protein interactions involved in the assembly of enzyme complexes, as with the 23/24 amino acid repeat in *C. thermocellum* mentioned earlier. Many polysaccharidases have a modular multiple domain structure consisting of catalytic and non-catalytic domains, or in a few cases, multiple catalytic domains (24).

CELLULASE GENES FROM RUMEN BACTERIA

Analyses of gene libraries from rumen bacteria made in bacteriophage vectors have revealed the existence of multiple genes encoding endoglucanases in the three main cellulolytic species (17, 20, 30). *F. succinogenes* S85 possesses at least nine different endoglucanase genes (20). It is not yet known how many different enzyme families are represented, but the two genes so far sequenced from different *F. succinogenes* strains belong to different families, A3 and E (20).

In the ruminococci a number of similar endoglucanase genes have been recovered from different strains. These encode relatively small products (350 to 450 amino acids) belonging to family A4 (10, 46, 49), although the cellulase gene isolated from *R. flavefaciens* 17 is now known to be larger than at first thought and clearly contains additional features (Flint *et al*, unp). A gene isolated from *R. flavefaciens* FD1 apparently encodes a cellodextrinase belonging to the A3 family (55). It seems possible that recovery of ruminococcal endoglucanase genes by cloning in plasmid vectors has been highly biased, however, since there is evidence that some sequences are unstable when present at high copy numbers in *E. coli* (49).

There are reports of bacterial and fungal 'avicelase' enzymes where a single gene product has high activity against crystalline cellulose (31, 61). So far no such exciting genes or enzymes have been isolated from rumen bacteria. Some of the cloned endoglucanases can degrade acid swollen cellulose, but avicelase activity is relatively low (20). It is not yet clear whether the ability to degrade crystalline cellulose is a function of several interacting gene products in rumen bacteria, or whether single genes encoding avicelase activity exist but have not yet been isolated. Synergy between isolated endoglucanases and exoglucanases from any one rumen bacterium with respect to the degradation of crystalline cellulose has not been reported. Synergy between enzyme preparations from *R. flavefaciens* and *B. fibrisolvens* has been reported, however, although the mechanism has not been elucidated (33).

A surprising feature of the cellulase and xylanase genes so far isolated from rumen bacteria, by comparison with other microorganisms (24) is that few have been shown to carry a substrate binding domain. It is possible that other, non-catalytic proteins are responsible for binding of an enzyme complex to the substrate, by analogy with *C. thermocellum*. In view of this there have been two cases in which binding domains from other bacteria have been deliberately added to rumen endoglucanases by gene fusion techniques. In one case this resulted in no significant change in functional properties (48), but in the other (38) some enhancement of the activity against crystalline cellulose was obtained.

XYLANASE GENES FROM RUMEN BACTERIA

Microbial xylanases belong mainly to two different enzyme families, F and G, although broad specificity endoglucanase/xylanase enzymes are also known that belong to family A (24). Family F xylanases have been reported from *B. fibrisolvens* (36, 40). In *R. flavefaciens* all three xylanase genes so far studied at the nucleotide sequence level are closely related at their amino terminal end, which encodes a family G xylanase. These genes therefore represent a family that appears to have arisen through successive gene duplications and fusions in evolution (Fig. 5.3). Two of the *R. flavefaciens* xylanase genes are known to encode products having two dissimilar catalytic domains, *XynA* having a family F xylanase as the carboxy terminal domain and *XynD* a β(1,3–1,4) glucanase (17, 62). This type of organisation is unusual, but has also been found previously in the non-rumen anaerobe *Caldocellum saccharolyticum* which encodes an exo/endo cellulase and an endoglucanase/mannanase each of which contain two distinct catalytic domains (22, 50). It also appears that the *XynC* gene of *F. succinogenes* encodes a xylanase containing two similar family

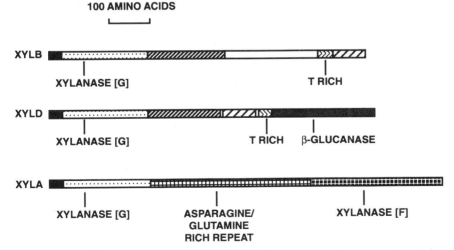

Figure 5.3. Multidomain xylanases of *Ruminococcus flavefaciens* 17. Regions having similar amino acid sequences are indicated with the same shading.

G xylanase domains (20), resembling in this respect a xylanase from the anaerobic fungus *Neocallimastix* (23).

Several possible explanations exist for the evolution of bifunctional polysaccharidases. On the one hand fusion of two distinct genes to produce a multifunctional polypeptide may simply provide a mechanism for coregulating expression that is the logical extension of the operon. In the case of polypeptides having similar domains, the duplication of coding regions might simply serve to boost expression. On the other hand it is tempting to think that bifunctional organisation may play a role in enhancing the catalytic efficiency of the enzyme. It might, for example, result in the release of oligosaccharides of a defined optimal size for uptake by the cell or processing by another enzyme. This would be a result of the precise juxtaposition of active sites, in contrast to the consequences of single domains acting randomly. It is not easy to see how this explanation would apply to the *R. flavefaciens* xylanase/β glucanase, however. Alternatively, dissimilar catalytic domains might interact synergistically in some way so as to enhance the hydrolysis of hemicellulosic matrix material. There is clearly scope for synergy between different hemicellulolytic activities in xylan breakdown (Fig. 5.1) (4), and synergy between arabinofuranosidase and xylanase activities has been demonstrated in *R. albus* (26).

Endoglucanase and xylanase genes so far isolated from different strains of *Prevotella ruminicola* have proved to belong to the same family of glycoside hydrolases (A) and presumably represent broad specificity enzymes that do not distinguish completely between the two substrates (20. 57). Recent work has shown that *P. ruminicola* strains also encode specific xylanases (Gasparic *et al*, unpublished).

DISTRIBUTION OF GENES IN DIFFERENT STRAINS

It is important to consider how widely the very detailed information that is obtained from gene isolation and sequencing applies to other genes or to other strains. We do not yet know precisely how many polysaccharidase genes having similar functions are present in any given rumen strain, nor how representative are the genes that have been cloned. DNA hybridisation methods have given some information on the distribution of cloned sequences between strains, however (Table 5.1). In *P. ruminicola* sequences resembling two cloned xylanase genes were found in strains closely related to the type strain 23, but there was

Table 5.1 INTER-STRAIN DISTRIBUTION OF SEQUENCES HYBRIDISING WITH CLONED POLYSACCHARIDASE GENES FROM RUMEN BACTERIA

Species	Gene used as probe:-			Strains surveyed by DNA hybridisation:-				
	Gene/ Plasmid	Encoded function	Strain of origin	Number	Number hybridising	Hybridis- ation stringency	Hybridising band patterns	Reference
Fibrobacter succinogenes	CelA	Endoglucanase	BL2	5	1 (+4)*	hi/lo	Different RF patterns in all strains	(19)
Butyrivibrio fibrisolvens	xynA	Xylanase (F)	49	13	3 (+6)*	hi/lo	2 strongly hybridizing strains gave same RF pattern	(40)
Prevotella ruminicola	pDDX1	Xylanase	D31d	26	3(+11)*	hi	Different RF patterns in all but 2 strains	(3)
	pRX30	Xylanase/ Endoglucanase (A)	23	26	6	hi	Different RF patterns in all strains	(3)
Ruminococcus albus	pTC1	Endoglucanase	AR67	2	1	hi		(58)
Ruminococcus flavefaciens	pMH1	Endoglucanase	AR68	2	1	hi		(58)
	xynA	Xylanase (G)	17	3	3	hi	Same 3.6Kb HindIII fragment	(19a)
		Xylanase (F)	17	2	2	hi	Same 3.6Kb HindIII fragment	(19a)

*(figures in brackets indicate strains giving weak hybridisation under stringent conditions)
[nb. Although cross-hybridisation is assumed to be due to polysaccharidase gene sequences, in many cases sequences flanking the gene were present in the DNA used for probing]

no hybridisation with other xylanolytic strains (3). In *F. succinogenes*, a cloned cellulase gene hybridised with DNA from all strains studied, but only under non-stringent conditions, indicating considerable DNA sequence divergence (19). In *R. albus* two endoglucanase genes isolated from different strains failed to cross-hybridise (56) and there is evidence of considerable interstrain divergence at the enzyme level (44). In contrast we have found that three *R. flavefaciens* strains, FD1, 17 and 007, all carry sequences related to the *xynA* gene of strain 17 on the same 3.6kb *Hind*III fragment (19a). In *B. fibrisolvens* a cloned family F xylanase showed an uneven distribution between strains which did not coincide with the phylogenetic relatedness of the strains (40).

In conclusion it is clear that strains of the same species can differ considerably in their complement and perhaps organisation of polysaccharidase genes, and that this variation may contribute to differences observed in the abilities of different strains to degrade plant cell wall material. On the other hand some of this variation may simply reflect sequence divergence between distantly related strains and need not imply functional divergence.

Conclusions

Much effort has gone into the initial characterisation of polysaccharidase genes from rumen bacteria in recent years. The challenge now is how to use this information to construct models for cell wall degradation by rumen bacteria and to understand the roles of individual gene products. This will require developing a more complete picture of the genes concerned, their expression and the interactions between their products in the host organism. Studying gene products expressed in *E. coli* has limitations. Large gene products are frequently subject to proteolytic breakdown (e.g. the *xynD* product of *R. flavefaciens* and the *cel 3* product of *F. succinogenes*); this has hindered investigations into the interactions of the two catalytic domains of *xynD*. In addition anomalous gene expression, e.g. due to the use of translational startpoints internal to the coding region, appears quite common. Furthermore the lack of posttranslational processing, e.g. glycosylation, may affect the properties of enzymes produced in *E. coli*. The ability to express cloned genes in alternative bacterial hosts more closely related to the original bacterium may prove helpful in resolving some of these problems. Furthermore improved techniques of gene transfer may create opportunities to study the roles of specific gene products in the original cellulolytic bacterium through enhancing or deliberately abolishing the expression of particular genes. At an ecological level it is clear that we are a long way from being able to identify the bacterial strains, let alone the gene products, that contribute most to plant cell wall degradation in the rumen. Various steps have been postulated that 'limit' fibre degradation. In such a complex system, however, it is very unlikely that any single factor will be identified as limiting the degradation of all forages under all conditions. Clearly under some conditions, and for some substrates, particular activities of the microbial cellulolytic population may be suboptimal, while under other conditions factors intrinsic to the structure of particular substrates may be more important. Much progress in understanding will come from testing the effects of enhancing particular microbial populations or activities; a few of these manipulations, at least, should enhance cell wall degradation under some conditions.

References

(1)   AKIN, D.E., BORNEMAN, W.S., RIGSBY, L.L. & MARTIN, S.A. (1993). *p*-coumaryl and feruloyl arabinoxylans from plant cell walls as substrates for ruminal bacteria. Appl. Environ. Microbiol. 59, 644–647.

(2)   AMANN, R.I., LIU, C., KAY, R., MONTGOMERY, L. & STAHL, D.A. (1992). Diversity among *Fibrobacter* isolates: towards a phylogenetic classification. Syst. Appl. Microbiol. 15, 23–31.

(3)   AVGUSTIN, G., FLINT, H.J. & WHITEHEAD, T.R. (1992). Distribution of xylanase genes and enzymes among strains of *Prevotella (Bacteroides) ruminicola* from the rumen. FEMS Microbiol. Lett., 99, 137–144.

(3a)   AVGUSTIN, G., WRIGHT, F.W. & FLINT, H.J. (1994) Genetic diversity and phylogenetic relationships among strains of *Prevotella (Bacteroides) ruminicola* from the rumen. Int. J. Syst. Bacteriol. 44, 246–255.

(4)   BIELY, P.C., MACKENZIE, G.R., PULS, J. & SCHNEIDER, H. (1986). Cooperativity of esterases and xylanase in the enzymatic degradation of acetyl xylan. Bio/Technol. 4, 731–733.

(5)   BRIESACHER, S.L., MAY, T., GRIGSBY, K.M., KERLEY, M.S., ANTHONY, R.V. & PATERSON, J.A. (1992). Uses of DNA probes to monitor nutritional effects on ruminal prokaryotes and *Fibrobacter succinogenes* S85. J. Anim. Sci. 70, 289–295.

(6)   CHENG, K-J., STEWART, C.S., DINSDALE, D. & COSTERTON, J.W. (1983/4). Electron microscopy of bacteria involved in the digestion of plant cell walls. Anim. Fd Sci. Technol. 10, 93–120.

(7)   CHESSON, A., FORSBERG, C.W. (1988). Polysaccharide degradation by rumen microorganisms In 'The Rumen Microbial Ecosystem'. P.N. Hobson (ed.) pp 257–284. Elsevier.

(8)   CHESSON, A. (1993). Mechanistic models of forage cell wall degradation In 'Forage Cell Wall Structure and Digestibility' H.G. Jung, D.R. Buxton, R.D. Hatfield and J. Ralph (ed.) pp 347–376. ASA-CSSA-SSSA Madison USA.

(9)   COUGHLAN, M.P. (1991). Mechanisms of cellulase degradation by fungi and bacteria. Anim. Fd Sci. Technol. 32, 77–100.

(10)   CUNNINGHAM, C., MCPHERSON, C.A., MARTIN, J., HARRIS, W.J. & FLINT, H.J. (1991). Sequence of a cellulase gene from the rumen anaerobe *Ruminococcus flavefaciens* 17. Mol. Gen. Genet. 228, 320–323.

(11)   DEHORITY, B.A. (1991). Effects of microbial synergism on fibre digestion in the rumen. Proc. Nutr. Soc. 50, 149–159.

(12)   DEHORITY, B.A. (1993). Microbial ecology of cell wall fermentation In 'Forage cell wall structure and digestibility' H.G. Jung, D.R. Buxton, R.D. Hatfield and J. Ralph (ed.) pp 425–453 ASA-CSSA-SSSA Madison USA.

(13)   DOERNER, K.C. & WHITE, B.A. (1990a). Assessment of the endo-1,4-β-glucanase components of *Ruminococcus flavefaciens* FD-1. Appl. Environ. Microbiol. 56, 1844–1850.

(14)   DOERNER, K.C. & WHITE, B.A. (1990b). Detection of glycoproteins separated by nondenaturing polyacrylamide gel electrophoresis using the periodic acid – Schiff stain. Anal. Biochem. 187, 147–150.

(15)   FLINT, H.J., MCPHERSON, C.A. & BISSET, J. (1989). Molecular cloning of genes from *Ruminococcus flavefaciens* encoding xylanase and β(1–3,1–4) glucanase activities. Appl. Environ. Microbiol. 55, 1230–1233.

(16)   FLINT, H. J. (1993). Molecular probes for studying changes in microbial populations in the gut. AFRC News, July 1993 p 10.

(17)   FLINT, H.J., MARTIN, J., MCPHERSON, M.C., DANIEL, A.S. & ZHANG, J-X. (1993). A bifunctional enzyme, with separate xylanase and β(1,3–1,4)-glucanase domains, encoded by the *xynD* gene of *Ruminococcus flavefaciens*. J. Bacteriol. 175, 2943–2951.

(18)   FLINT, H.J., MCPHERSON, M.C. & MARTIN, J. (1991). Expression of two xylanase genes from the rumen cellulolytic bacterium *Ruminococcus flavefaciens* 17 cloned in pUC13. J. Gen. Microbiol. 137, 123–129.

(19)   FLINT, H.J., MCPHERSON, C.A., AVGUSTIN, G. & STEWART, C.S. (1990). Use of a cellulase encoding gene probe to reveal restriction fragment length polymorphisms among ruminal strains of *Bacteroides succinogenes*. Curr. Microbiol. 20, 63–67.

(19a)   FLINT, H.J., McPHERSON, C.A., ZHANG, J-X., MARTIN, J., GARCIA-CAMPAYO, V. AND WOOD, T.M. (1994). Relationships of xylanase genes from rumen bacteria. In Genetics, Biochemistry and Ecology of Lignocellulose Degradation. (Shimada, K., Hoshino, S., Ohmiya, K., Sakka, K., Kobayashi, Y. & Karita, S. eds) pp. 188–196. Uni Publishers, Tokyo.

(20)   FORSBERG, C.W., CHENG, K-J., KRELL, P.J. & PHILLIPS, J.P. (1993). Establishment of rumen microbial genepools and their manipulation to benefit fibre degradation by domestic animals. pp 281–316 Vol 1, Proc. VIIth Wld Conf. Anm. Prod.

(21)   GARDNER, R.M., DOERNER, K.C. & WHITE, B.A. (1987). Purification and characterization of an exo-β-1,4-glucanase from *Ruminococcus flavefaciens* FD-1. J. Bacteriol. 169, 4581–4588.

(22)   GIBBS, M.D., SAUL, D.J., LUTHI, E. & BERGQUIST, P.L. (1992). The β-mannanase from '*Caldocellum saccharolyticum*' is part of a multidomain enzyme. Appl. Environ. Microbiol. 58, 3864–3867.

(23)   GILBERT, H.J., HAZLEWOOD, G.P., LAURIE, J.I. ORPIN, C.G. & XUE, G.P. (1992). Homologous catalytic domains in a rumen fungal xylanase: evidence for gene duplication and prokaryotic origin. Mol. Microbiol. 6, 2065–2076.

(24)   GILKES, N.R., HENRISSAT, D.G., KILBURN, D.G., MILLER, R.C. & WARREN, R.A.J. (1991). Domains in microbial β-1,4-glycanases: sequence conservation, function and enzyme families. Microbiol. Rev. 55, 303–315.

(25) GREVE, L.C., LABAVITCH, J.M., STACK, R.J., HUNGATE, R.E. (1984a). Muralytic activities of *Ruminococcus albus* 8. Appl. Environ. Microbiol. 47, 1141–1145.

(26) GREVE, L.C., LABAVITCH, J.M. & HUNGATE, R.E. (1984b). α-L-arabinofuranosidase from *Ruminococcus albus* 8: purification and possible role in hydrolysis of alfalfa cell wall. Appl. Env. Microbiol. 47, 1135–1140.

(27) HALLIWELL, G. & BRYANT, M.D. (1963). The cellulolytic activity of pure strains of bacteria from the rumen of cattle. J. Gen. Microbiol. 32, 441–448.

(28) HATFIELD, R.D. (1993). Cell wall polysaccharide interactions and degradability In 'Forage Cell Wall Structure and Digestibility' H.G. Jung, D.R. Buxton, R.D. Hatfield and J. Ralph (ed) pp 285–313 ASA-CSSA-SSSA. Madison USA.

(29) HESPELL, R.B. & O'BRYAN-SHAH, P.J. (1988). Esterase activity in *Butyrivibrio fibrisolvens* strains. Appl. Environ. Microbiol. 54, 1917–1922.

(30) HOWARD, G.T. & WHITE, B.A. (1988). Molecular cloning and expression of cellulase genes from *Ruminococcus albus* 8 in *Escherichia coli* bacteriophage λ. Appl. Environ. Microbiol. 54, 1752–1755.

(31) JAURIS, S., RUCKNAGEL, K.P. SCHWARTZ, W.H., DRATSCH, P., BRONNENMEIER, K. & STAUDENBAUER, W.L. (1990). Sequence analysis of the *Clostridium stercorarium cfIz* gene encoding a thermoactive cellulase (Avicelase I): identification of catalytic and cellulose binding domains. Mol. Gen. Genet 223, 258–267.

(32) KOHRING, S., WIEGEL, J. & MAYER, F. (1990). Subunit composition and glycosidic activities of the cellulase complex from *Clostridium thermocellum* JW20. Appl. Env. Microbiol, 56 (12), 3798–3804.

(33) KOPECNY, J. & WILLIAMS, A.G.(1988). Synergism of rumen microbial hydrolases and degradation of plant polymers. Folia Microbiol. 33, 208–212.

(34) LAMED, R., NAIMARK, J., MORGENSTERN, E. & BAYER, E.A. (1987). Specialized cell surface structures in cellulolytic bacteria. J. Bacteriol. 169, 3792–3800.

(35) LIN, L.L. & THOMSON, J.A. (1991). An analysis of the extracellular cellulases and xylanases of *Butyrivibrio fibrisolvens* H17c. FEMS Micro Letters 84, 197–204.

(36) LIN, L.L. & THOMSON, J.A. (1991). Cloning, sequencing and expression of a gene encoding a 73KDa xylanase enzyme from the rumen anaerobe *Butyrivibrio fibrisolvens* H17c. Mol. Gen. Genet. 228, 55–61.

(37) McDERMID K.P., MacKENZIE, C.R. & FORSBERG, C.W. (1990). Esterase activites of *Fibrobacter succinogenes* subsp. *succinogenes* S85. Appl. Environ. Microbiol. 56, 127–132.

(38) MAGLIONE, G.R., MATSUSHITA, O., RUSSELL, J.B. & WILSON, D.B. (1992). Properties of a genetically reconstructed *Prevotella ruminicola* endoglucanase. Appl. Env. Microbiol. 58, 3593–3597.

(39) MANNARELLI, B.M. (1988). Deoxyribonucleic acid relatedness among strains of the species *Butyrivibrio fibrisolvens*. Int. J. Syst. Bacteriol. 38, 340–347.

(40) MANNARELLI, B.M., EVANS, S. & LEE, D. (1990). Cloning, sequencing and expression of a xylanase gene from the anaerobic ruminal bacterium *Butyrivibrio fibrisolvens*. J. Bacteriol 172,4247–4254.

(41) MANNARELLI, B.M., ERICSSON, L.D., LEE, D., STACK, R.J. (1991). Taxonomic relationshps among strains of the anaerobic bacterium *Bacteroides ruminicola* determined by DNA and extracellular polysaccharide analysis. Appl. Environ. Microbiol. 57, 2975–2980.

(42) MORAG, E., HALEVY, I., BAYER, E.A. & LAMED, R. (1991). Isolation and properties of a major cellobiohydrolase from the cellulosome of *Clostridium thermocellum*. J. Bacteriol. 173 (13), 4155–4162.

(43) MORRIS, E.J. & VAN GYLSWYK, N.O. (1980). Comparison of the action of rumen bacteria on cell walls from *Eragrostis tef*. J. Agric. Sci. Camb. 95, 313–323.

(44) MORRIS, E.J. & COLE, O.J. (1987). Relationship between cellulolytic activity and adhesion to cellulose in *Ruminococcus albus*. J. Gen. Microbiol. 133, 1023–1032.

(45) OHMIYA, K., SHIMIZU, M., TAYA, M. & SHIMIZA, S. (1982). Purification and properties of a cellobiosidase from *Ruminococcus albus*. J. Bacteriol. 150, 407–407.

(46) OHMIYA, K., KAJINO, T., KATO, A. & SHIMIZU, S. (1989). Structure of a *Ruminococcus albus* endo-1,4,-β-glucanase gene. J. Bacteriol. 171, 6771–6775.

(47) PETTIPHER, G.L. & LATHAM, M.J. (1979). Characteristics of enzymes produced by *Ruminococcus flavefaciens* which degrade plant cell walls. J. Gen. Microbiol. 110, 21–27.

(48)   POOLE, D.H., DURRANT, A.J., HAZLEWOOD, G.P. & GILBERT, H.J. (1991). Characterisation of hybrid proteins consisting of the catalytic domains of *Clostridium* and *Ruminococcus* endoglucanses, fused to *Pseudomonas* non-catlaytic cellulose binding domains. Biochem. J. 279, 787–792.

(49)   POOLE, D.M., HAZLEWOOD, G.P., LEWIS, J.I., BARKER, P.J. & GILBERT, H.J. (1990). Nucleotide sequence of the *Ruminococcus albus* SY3 endoglucanase genes *celA* and *celB*. Mol. Gen. Genet. 223, 217–223.

(50)   SAUL, D.J., WILLIAMS, L.C., GRAYLING, R.A., CHAMLEY, L.W., LOVE, D.R. & BERGQUIST, P.L. (1990). *celA*, a gene coding for a bifunctional cellulase from the extreme thermophile '*Caldocellum saccharolyticum*'. Appl. Env. Microbiol. 56, 3117–3124.

(51)   STAHL, D.A., FLESHER, D., MANSFIELD, H.R. & MONTGOMERY, L. (1988). Use of phylogenetically based hybridisation probes for studies of ruminal microbial ecology. Appl. Environ. Microbiol. 54, 1079–1084.

(52)   STEWART, C.S. & BRYANT, M.P. (1988). The rumen bacteria In 'The Rumen Microbial Ecosystem' P.N. Hobson (ed.) pp 21–75 Elsevier Applied Sciences, London.

(53)   STEWART, C.S., DUNCAN, S.H., MCPHERSON, C.A., RICHARDSON, A.J. & FLINT, H.J. (1990). The implications of the loss and regain of cotton-degrading activity for the degradation of straw by *Ruminococcus flavefaciens* 007. J.Appl. Bacteriol. 68, 349–356.

(54)   VAN GYLSWYK, N.O. & SCHWARTZ, H.M. (1984). Microbial ecology of the rumen of animals fed high fibre diets. pp. 359–377 In Herbivore Nutrition in the Subtropics and Tropics ed Gilchrist, F.M.C and Mackie, R.I. Science Press Ltd SA.

(55)   WANG, W. & THOMSON, J.A. (1992). Nucleotide sequence of the *celA* gene encoding a cellodextrinase of *Ruminococcus flavefaciens* FD1. Mol. Gen. Genet. 233, 492.

(56)   WARE, G.E., BAUCHOP, T. & GREGG, K. (1989). The isolation and comparison of cellulase genes from two strains of *Ruminococcus albus*. J. Gen. Microbiol. 135, 921–930.

(57)   WHITEHEAD, T.R. (1993). Analyses of gene and amino acid sequence of the *Prevotella (Bacteroides) ruminicola* 23 xylanase reveals unexpected homology with endoglucanases from other genera of bacteria. Curr. Microbiol. 27, 27–33.

(58) WONG, K.K.Y., TAN, L.U.L. & SADDLER, J.N. (1988). Multiplicity of β-1,4-xylanase in microorganisms: functions and applications. Microbiol. Rev. 52, 305–317.

(59) WOOD, T.M. & MACRAE, S.I. (1979). Synergism between enzymes involved in the solubilization of native cellulose. In Adv. Chem. Ser. 181 ed. R.D. Brown Jr. and L. Jurasek. Amer. Chem. Soc. Washington pp 181–210.

(60) WOOD, T.M., WILSON, C.A. & STEWART, C.S. (1982). Preparation of the cellulase from the cellulolytic rumen bacterium *Ruminococcus albus* and its release from the bacterial cell wall. Biochem. J. 205, 129–137.

(61) XUE, G.P., ORPIN, C.G., GOBIUS, K.S., AYLWARD, J.H. & SIMPSON, G.D. (1992). Cloning and expression of multiple cellulase cDNAs from the anaerobic fungus *Neocallimastix patriciarum* in *Escherichia coli*. J. Gen Microbiol. 138, 1413–1420.

(62) ZHANG, J-X. & FLINT, H.J. (1992). A bifunctional xylanase encoded by the *xynA* gene of the rumen cellulolytic bacterium *Ruminococcus flavefaciens* 17 comprises two dissimilar domains linked by an asparagine/glutamine rich sequence. Mol. Microbiol. 6, 1013–1023

6

PLANT CELL-WALL DEGRADATION BY RUMEN PROTOZOA

J.P. JOUANY[1] and K. USHIDA[2]
[1]Unité de la Digestion Microbienne, Centre de Recherches de Clermont Ferrand-Theix, 63122 Saint Genès-Champanelle, France
[2]Kyoto Prefectural University, Shimogamo, Kyoto, 606 Japan

Summary

Although the presence of protozoa in the rumen is generally considered to improve cell wall carbohydrate degradation, the reverse effect has been observed by different authors. These apparent discrepancies are explained by the diverse targets the protozoa have in the rumen and their respective importance. Examples will be given to illustrate how protozoa can have opposite effects on cellulolysis in the rumen (interaction with starch, level of ammonia-nitrogen concentration). The qualitative composition of the fauna, which is greatly influenced by the diet, can also modulate the action of protozoa against plant cell walls. A recent experiment with isolated genera of protozoa (*Polyplastron*, *Eudiplodinium*, *Epidinium*, *Entodinium*, *Isotricha*) is presented to show their different abilities to digest and ferment various kinds of pure celluloses. We also showed that large ciliate protozoa are more effective against the hemicellulose fraction than the cellulose fraction.

Introduction

Although many studies have been made to determine the effect of the presence or the absence of ciliates in the rumen since the work of Becker *et al* in 1929 (2), there is still debate among scientists concerning the real impact of protozoa on cell-wall carbohydrate digestion in ruminants (3, 9). Nor is the direct contribution of protozoa in rumen cell-wall digestion fully known. This can be explained by the numerous factors involved in cellulolysis, which can be altered by the presence of proto-

69

zoa: cellulolytic activity of rumen microbes (specific activity of proto-zoa, interactions with bacteria and fungi), and physical or physiological factors such as colonization (rate, extent), environmental conditions (pH, VFA composition, N-NH3 concentration) and reten-tion time in the rumen. All these aspects must be considered to explain the overall effect of rumen protozoa in the digestion of forages. In addition, protozoa should not be considered as a uniform group since the different genera have specific digestive abilities, as shown for protein degradation (10). In the future, it is likely that the specificity of each genus will be used to improve feed efficiency in ruminant produc-tion by controlling the composition of the rumen fauna.

Some original results are presented in this paper to characterize the ability to digest plant cell walls of the major ciliate genera. Novel explanations are suggested for the converse responses of the same protozoa obtained in the cell wall digestive experiments.

Direct contribution of rumen protozoa in plant cell wall digestion

DEGRADATION AND FERMENTATION OF DIFFERENT CELLULOSIC SUBSTRATES BY VARIOUS CILIATE GENERA

It has been estimated from calculations and assumptions that a quarter to one-third of fiber breakdown in the rumen is of protozoal origin (1, 5, 14, 18). It is known that large entodiniomorphid protozoa contain a range of enzymes that are active against plant structural carbohydrates (4, 17). The ability of holotrichs to degrade plant cell wall carbo-hydrates (cellulose, hemicellulose) is much more limited. They have low depolymerizing activity against ryegrass hemicellulose and oat xylan, but do not ferment the formed products. The reported findings on the presence of holotrich β-glucanase are inconclusive.

Using pure genera of protozoa, to which antibiotics had been added in 24-hr incubations to eliminate cellulolytic bacteria, we tested the degradation of 4 types of pure cell wall polymeric carbohydrates [highly-crystalline cellulose (Avicel), 2 substituted celluloses (HEC and CMC), and oat xylan] by *Eudiplodinium*, *Polyplastron*, *Epidinium*, *Entodinium*, *Isotricha*. The products of fermentation and the growth of protozoa were also determined and quantified.

There are great differences between genera in the ability of Ophryos-

Table 6.1 DEGRADATION OF PURE SUBSTRATES BY ISOLATED AND DECONTAMINATED PROTOZOAL CULTURES (24 hrs).

Substrates protozoa	Avicel (%)*	HEC (%)+	CMC (%)+	Xylan
Eudiplodinium	24.9 ± 7.8	62.0 ± 3.8	62.8 ± 0.7	ND
Polyplastron	30.6 ± 2.9	55.2 ± 5.5	60.3 ± 1.3	ND
Epidinium	10.0 ± 2.7	62.3 ± 0.9	63.7 ± 2.6	ND
Entodinium	trace	28.7 ± 1.7	22.7 ± 1.1	ND
Isotricha	5.4 ± 1.7	54.1 ± 0.8	42.3 ± 3.9	ND

ND: not determined; HEC: hexa ethyl cellulose; CMC: carboxy methyl cellulose.
*n = 6; +n = 4

colecids to degrade crystalline cellulose (Avicel). *Eudiplodinium* and *Polyplastron* were both able to hydrolyse 30% of avicel in our 24-hr incubations (Table 6.1). *Epidinium* degradation accounted for only 10%, while *Entodinium* had no effect. Only a slight action of *Isotricha* against Avicel was detected.

Nearly 60% of substituted celluloses (HEC, CMC) disappeared in presence of the large Ophryoscolecids (*Eudiplodinium, Polyplastron, Epidinium*), while only 25% were degraded in the presence of *Entodinium* (Table 6.1); *Isotricha* had an intermediate ability (50% degradation).

The use by protozoa of the products obtained from the hydrolysis of the substrates was estimated through VFA and gas productions, and the growth of protozoa during incubations. *Eudiplodinium* and *Polyplastron* had similar fermentation activities (Table 6.2). They used xylan as a source of energy at half the rate of that of starch; fermentations from Avicel were four fold less active than those from xylan, but

Table 6.2 VFA AND GAS PRODUCTIONS (μmoles and ml/1000 ciliates).

	Substrates:	Starch#	Avicel*	Xylan+	HEC+	CMC+
Eudiplodinium	VFA	4350	712	2225	0	0
	gas	13.7	1.9	3.1	0	0
Polyplastron	VFA	2725	875	2275	0	0
	gas	7.2	1.2	3.7	0	0
Epidinium	VFA	407	50	225	0	0
	gas	1.0	0.1	0.6	0	0
Entodinium	VFA	325	11	26	25	37
	gas	0.5	0	0	0	0
Isotricha	VFA	14416	0	ND	0	0
	gas	10.0	0	0	0	0

ND = not determined; HEC: hexa ethyl cellulose; CMC: carboxy methyl cellulose.
#n = 10; *n = 6; +n = 4
Incubations were fed with 80 mg of substrates

did not use the substituted celluloses. *Epidinium* had a lower rate of fermentation for all the substrates tested (five to ten fold lower than *Eudiplodinium* and *Polyplastron*). Compared to the large Ophroscolecids, the small Entodinia had a low fermentative activity with the substrates tested. However, if comparisons were made on the same biomass basis, the use of substrates by Entodinia would be greatly improved. *Entodinium* seems to have some ability to ferment the products from hydrolysis of substituted celluloses.

Compared to the negative-control incubations to which no substrate was added, and to the positive-control incubations which were fed with starch, the growth of *Eudiplodinium* was high in the presence of Avicel and xylan (Table 6.3). *Polyplastron* also used Avicel and xylan for growth, but to a lesser extent. *Epidinium* had particularly high growth with xylan as energy source but used little Avicel. *Entodinium* used none of the substrates tested. *Isotricha* maintained growth even in the negative-control incubations and in the presence of the cell-wall substrates tested, while its population increased two fold when starch was added.

This experiment shows that there are great differences between protozoa in their ability to hydrolyse cell-wall carbohydrates and to use them as energy source. This means that not only the number of protozoa has to be considered in the rumen, but also the qualitative composition of the ciliate population.

The three large Ophryoscolecids tested were all active against xylan and used it for growth. Only *Eudiplodinium* and *Polyplastron* degraded and used crystalline cellulose. They all degraded substituted celluloses but were unable to use the products formed during hydrolysis. Small Entodinia were not effective against the substrates tested. *Isotricha* had a slight β-glucanase activity but were not able to use the products for growth.

Table 6.3   NUMBER OF LIVING PROTOZOA AT THE END OF 24 h INCUBATIONS (% OF THE NUMBER AT THE START OF INCUBATIONS)

	Control[+]	*Starch*[+]	*Avicel*[*]	*Xylan*[*]	*HEC*[#]	*CMC*[#]
Eudiplodinium	<5	401	147	200	<5	<5
Polyplastron	34	85	58	60	20	15
Epidinium	6	12	9	100	<50	<5
Entodinium	<5	<5	<5	<5	<5	<5
Isotricha	95	181	89	77	94	103

Control: no substrate was added to incubations
[+]n = 10; [*]n = 6; [#]n = 4

Table 6.4   INFLUENCE OF PROTOZOA ON RUMINAL DIGESTION OF CELL WALL COMPONENTS (FROM BIBLIOGRAPHIC DATA)

Diet	Digestion of hemicellulose (%)		Digestion of cellulose (%)		Authors
	Defaunated	Faunated	Defaunated	Faunated	
Lucerne (66) + barley (31) + straw (3)	33.2[a]	57.7[b]	31.5[a]	41.0[b]	Ushida and Jouany (1990)
NaOH straw (70) + Beet pulp (16) + soya (14)	37.9[a]	52.9[b]	54.4[a]	58.0[b]	"
NH_3 straw (93) + fishmeal (7):	60.3[a]	72.0[b]	62.8	65.5	Ushida *et al* (1990)
xylose	62.5	69.7	glucose: 64.5	68.5	"
mannose + galactose	73.9	81.5			"
arabinose	72.5	79.2			"
NH_3 straw (73) + maize (20) + fishmeal (7)	26.8[a]	57.6[b]	51.3[a]	66.2[b]	"
xylose	42.6[a]	64.7[b]	glucose: 42.7[a]	60.2[b]	"
mannose + galactose	38.9[a]	62.9[b]			"
arabinose	61.1[a]	69.9[b]			"

a, b, means followed by different letters were significantly different ($p \leq 0.05$)

DO PROTOZOA HAVE A SPECIFIC ROLE IN CELL WALL CARBOHYDRATE DEGRADATION?

Few *in vivo* studies using duodenal fistulated animals have been made to characterize the effect of protozoa on the digestion of the different components of plant cell walls. Table 6.4 shows that the addition of protozoa to a defaunated rumen increases both cellulose and hemicellulose digestion. However, this increase is always far greater in the hemicellulosic fraction. Although the differences between defaunated and faunated animals cannot be attributed solely to the function of protozoa, the concordance of the results and the amplitude of the effect can be related to the high xylanase activity of large Ophryoscolecids we showed previously.

The plant cell wall components are assembled in a complex network that strengthens the cell wall architecture and provides great resistance to the chemical and biological agents. In *Graminae*, hemicelluloses are linked to lignin by covalent chemical bonds in which arabinose, uronic acids and hydroxycinnamic acids are involved, but there are no direct linkages between lignin and cellulose (Figure 6.1). Cellulose is closely

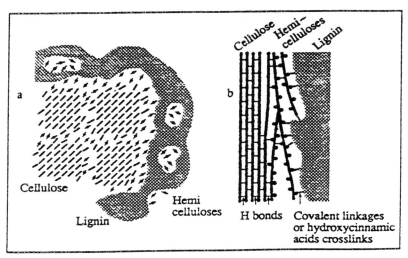

Figure 6.1. Model of the association of cell wall components (from (6))

associated to hemicellulose by chemical linkages. The positive action of rumen protozoa on cell wall digestion is probably due to their hydrolytic activity against hemicellulose by separating lignin from some of the potential degradable carbohydrates, which makes them more readily available to the microbial enzymes. Such an action would theoretically increase the amount of lignin-carbohydrate complexes produced in the rumen.

The effect of dietary interactions on the response of protozoa in cell wall degradation

EFFECT OF THE PRESENCE OF STARCH IN DIETS

Measurements of the duodenal flow in faunated and defaunated fistulated sheep have shown lignocellulose digestion by protozoa is enhanced when the diet is supplemented with starch (16). This suggests that there are interactions between dietary starch, the presence of protozoa, and the digestion of cell wall components. These interactions probably differ according to the protozoa. Thus, the substitution of 20% straw by maize in a NH_3-treated straw-based diet increased the positive effect of protozoa on lignocellulose digestion (+114 and +29% vs +20% and +4% respectively for hemicellulose and cellulose rumen digestibilities).

Because of a high uptake of starch granules and starch-associated bacteria, the concentration of amylolytic and lactic bacteria decreased when protozoa were present (12, 13). This means that defaunated animals are more sensitive to the risk of acidosis. Lactic acid concentration and pH levels were therefore more favourable to the growth of cellulolytic bacteria in faunated than in the defaunated animals. Protozoa may favour the growth of fungi since the latter are sensitive to high acidic conditions (7), but there are no published results to support this.

Probably for the same reasons, it has been reported that the inoculation of *Entodinium*, a non cellulolytic protozoa, in a defaunated rumen improved lignocellulose digestion when large amounts of readily fermentable carbohydrate were supplemented, while it failed to improve digestion when a 100% grass hay diet was fed (8). These diet-dependent effects of *Entodinium* were further confirmed *in vitro* (11).

The results of the degradation of wheat straw *in sacco* (Figure 6.2) show that the presence of starch sometimes give an advantage to defaunated animals. These means that other factors must be considered to understand the real impact of protozoa on rumen cell wall digestion.

EFFECT OF THE RUMEN AMMONIA CONCENTRATION

It is now known that defaunation decreases rumen ammonia concentration as the result of a lower deamination during protein degradation and a higher uptake of ammonia by a larger bacterial population, and a smaller recycling of microbial proteins. Thus, two situations can be considered: 1) Either the concentration of ammonia nitrogen is just enough to give the highest degradation of cell walls in faunated animals; in this case there will be a NH_3-N shortage in defaunated animals and, as a consequence, the cell wall carbohydrate digestion will be decreased. Or, the supply of dietary soluble nitrogen is much higher than necessary for both faunated and defaunated animals; the NH_3-N concentration will be above the minimum required for optimization of cellulolysis. If this is so, cellulolysis will be optimal in defaunated animals fed on poor roughages not supplemented with starch. *In vitro*, the relation between ammonia concentration and the response of animals to defaunation has been demonstrated (15). Protozoa can therefore be considered as a promoter of ammonia formation, which is a disadvantage for nitrogen utilization, but is favourable to cell wall degradation when animals are fed on diets with a high ratio of

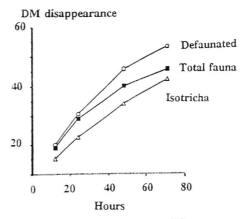

Diet: grass hay (70) + barley (30)
Amount: 1200 g d⁻¹ fed continuously

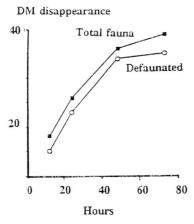

Diet: NH₃ wheat straw (94) +
fishmeal (6).
Amount: 900 g d⁻¹ fed continuously

Diet: dehydrated lucerne (60) +
barley (26) + grass hay/wheat
straw (14)
Amount: 1150 g d⁻¹ fed once daily

Figure 6.2. Effect of protozoa on the *in situ* degradation of wheat straw in sheep fed different diets.

energy/soluble nitrogen. This hypothesis needs to be confirmed by specially designed *in vivo* experiments.

Depending on feeding conditions and the nutritional needs of animals, protozoa can be considered either as parasites or as symbionts. Their action in the rumen can vary according to animals and diets, and for this reason more precise studies should be made on the effect of the different ciliate genera on rumen functions.

References

(1)   AMOS, H.E. and AKIN, D.E. (1978). Rumen protozoal degradation of structurally intact forage tissues. Applied and Environmental Microbiology 36, 513–522.

(2)   BECKER, E.R., SCHULZ, J.A. and EMMERSON, M.A. (1929). Experiments on the physiological relationships between the stomach infusoria of ruminants and their hosts, with a bibliography. Journal of Science 64, 215–251.

(3)   BIRD, S. and LENG, R.A. (1984). Further studies on the effects of the presence or absence of protozoa in the rumen on liveweight gain and wool growth in sheep. British Journal of Nutrition 52, 607–611.

(4)   COLEMAN, G.S. (1985). The cellulase content of 15 species of entodiniomorphid protozoa, mixed bacteria and plant debris isolated from the ovine rumen. Journal of Agricultural Science, Cambridge 104, 349–360.

(5)   DEMEYER, D.I. (1981). Rumen microbes and digestion of plant cell walls. Agriculture and Environment 6, 295–337.

(6)   FENGEL, D. and WEGENER, G. (1984). Wood: chemistry, ultrastructure, reactions, (Walter de Gruyter ed.), Springer Verlag, Berlin, 613 pages.

(7)   GRENET, E., BRETON, A., BARRY, P. and FONTY, G. (1989). Rumen anaerobic fungi and plant substrates colonization as affected by diet composition. Animal Feed Science and Technology 26, 55–70.

(8)   JOUANY, J.P. and SENAUD, J. (1983). Influence des ciliés du rumen sur la digestion de différents glucides chez le mouton. 1 Utilisation des glucides pariétaux (cellulose et hémicelluloses) et de l'amidon. Reproduction, Nutrition et Développement 22, 735–752.

(9)   JOUANY, J.P., DEMEYER, D.I. and GRAIN, J. (1988). Effect of defaunating the rumen.Animal Feed Science and Technology 21, 229–265.

(10) JOUANY, J.P., IVAN, M., PAPON, Y. and LASSALAS, B (1992). Effects of *Isotricha, Eudiplodinium+ Entodinium* and a mixed population of rumen protozoa on the *in vitro* degradation

of fish meal, soybean meal and casein. Canadian Journal of Animal Science 72, 871–880.

(11)   KANEKO, T., USHIDA, K. and KOJIMA, Y. (1989). Effect of starch on cellulolysis by rumen microbial populations with or without protozoa. In: *The Role of Protozoa and Fungi in Ruminant Digestion* (Nolan, J.V., Leng, R.A. and Demeyer, D.I. eds.) pp. 313–315. Perambul Books, Armidale, Australia.

(12)   KURIHARA, Y., EADIE, J.M., HOBSON, P.N. and MANN, S.O. (1968). Relationship between bacteria and ciliate protozoa in the sheep rumen. Journal of General Microbiology 51, 267–287.

(13)   KURIHARA, Y., TAKECHI, T. and SHIBATA, F. (1978). Relationship between bacteria and ciliate protozoa in the rumen of sheep fed on a purified diet. Journal of Agricultural Science, Cambridge 90, 373–381.

(14)   LUBBERDING, H.J., GIJZEN, H.J., GERHARDUS, M.J. and VOGELS, G.D. (1987). Fibre degradation and activities in an artificial rumen system in the presence and the absence of rumen ciliates. In: *Physiology of Ruminant Nutrition*, (Boda, K. ed.) pp 127–135. Slovak Academy of Sciences, Kosice, Czekoslovakia.

(15)   USHIDA, K. and KOJIMA, Y. (1991). Effect of defaunation and refaunation of the rumen on cellulolytic activity *in vitro* with or without ammonia supplementation. Canadian Journal of Animal Science 71, 913–917.

(16)   USHIDA, K., KAYOULI, C., DE SMET, S. and JOUANY, J.P. (1990). Effect of defaunation on protein and fibre digestion in sheep fed on ammonia-treated straw-based diets with and without maize. British Journal of Nutrition 64, 765–775.

(17)   WILLIAMS, A.G. and COLEMAN, G.S. (1985). Hemicellulose degrading enzymes in rumen ciliate protozoa. Current Microbiology 12, 85–90.

(18)   WILLIAMS, A.G. and STRACHAN, N.H. (1984). The distribution of polysaccharide-degrading enzymes in the bovine digesta ecosystem. Current Microbiology 10, 215–220.

7

ANAEROBIC FUNGI, THEIR DISTRIBUTION AND LIFE CYCLE

A.P.J. TRINCI[1], A. RICKERS[1], K. GULL[1], D.R. DAVIES[1], B.B. NIELSEN[1,2], W.Y. ZHU[2] and M.K. THEODOROU[2]
[1]*School of Biological Sciences, Stopford Building, University of Manchester, Manchester, M13 9PT, U.K.*
[2]*AFRC Inst. of Grassland & Environmental Research, Plas Gogerddan, Aberystwyth, Dyfed, SY23 3EB, U.K.*

Summary

Anaerobic fungi have been isolated world wide (from at least 16 countries) from foregut-fermenting (31 animal species) and hindgut-fermenting (9 animal species) herbivores. For cattle, they have been isolated from each part of the digestive tract, and, for sheep, from both fresh and dried (stored for up to 10 months) faeces. Transfer of anaerobic fungi between animals may occur via aerosols, saliva or faeces, with the latter probably containing resistant structures such as cysts or resistant zoosporangia. To date 13 species of anaerobic fungi have been described, all of which are classified in the Order Neocallimasticales of the Class Chytridiomycetes (True Fungi). Like other members of this class, they form either monocentric or polycentric thalli. The use of monoclonal and polyclonal antibodies to detect different stages of the life cycle will be described, and the use of gas pressure as an indicator of the growth of batch cultures of anaerobic fungi will be discussed.

Geographical distribution of anaerobic fungi

Since their first isolation in the U.K. from the rumen of sheep (45) anaerobic fungi have been isolated from animals in Australia (53), (34); Canada (33); Chile (Dr. M.K. Theodorou and Dr. W.Y. Zhu; unpublished result); Czechoslovakia (44); Ethiopia (41); France (15); Holland (54); Indonesia (Dr. M.K. Theodorou; personal communication); Japan (60); Malaysia (22), (23), (34); New Zealand (6), (7); Norway

(49); Russia (32); Tanzania (11) and U.S.A. (1). It would appear, therefore, that anaerobic fungi have a world wide distribution.

Distribution of anaerobic fungi amongst herbivores

The discovery that it is possible to isolate anaerobic fungi from faeces (39) provided a simple way of surveying herbivores for these organisms. To date they have been isolated from 31 foregut-fermenting herbivores and 9 hindgut-fermenting herbivores (59). Thus, anaerobic fungi are ubiquitous amongst herbivores. However, anaerobic fungi have not been isolated from habitats other than the digestive tract of herbivorous mammals and their faeces; attempts to isolate them from mud and from landfill sites have proved unsuccessful (51), (55).

Transfer of anaerobic fungi between animals

Lowe *et al.* (39) isolated anaerobic fungi from saliva taken from sheep and Milne *et al.* (41) showed that anaerobic fungi survived for up to 8 h in sheep saliva stored in air at 39°C. Thus, like bacteria (30), anaerobic fungi may be dispersed between ruminants in aerosols formed from saliva. Anaerobic fungi have been isolated from fresh faeces (39) and dried faeces stored in air for a number of months (41), (56). In the aerobic chytrids, resistant structures are formed following sexual reproduction, or by the formation of resistant zoosporangia or cysts (31). However, the occurrence of such structures in anaerobic fungi has not been confirmed, although the isolation of anaerobic fungi from air-dried faeces of both foregut- and hindgut-fermenting herbivores suggests they probably exist (41), (56), (13). After drying, populations of anaerobic fungi in faeces decline very slowly and isolations can still be made for up to 10 months after the onset of drying (41), (56). Anaerobic fungi have even been isolated in Ethiopia from sun-baked dung of cattle and sheep (41). Zoosporangia of anaerobic fungi have been observed on digesta particles recovered from cow faeces and these digesta particles have been shown to give rise to cultures of anaerobic fungi (Ms. B.B. Nielsen, Prof. A.P.J. Trinci & Dr. M.K. Theodorou, unpublished result). Thus, faeces may serve as a route for transfer of anaerobic fungi between herbivores: ruminants are not coprophagic but accidental contact with fresh or dried faeces may occur.

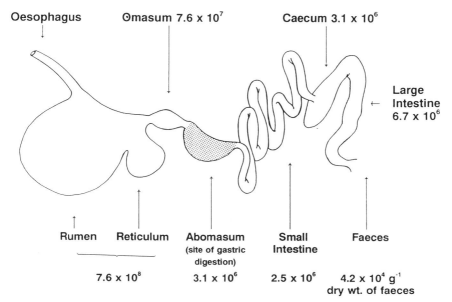

Figure 7.1. Estimates of the *total* number of thallus forming units of anaerobic fungi in each part of the digestive tract of cattle and the *concentration* of anaerobic fungi in faeces [from (13)]

Distribution of anaerobic fungi within the digestive tract

By using a most probable number procedure and by determining the amount of digesta in each organ, Davies *et al.* (13) were able to enumerate populations of anaerobic fungi in the digestive tract and faeces of cattle (Fig. 7.1). These results suggest the presence of a resistant stage in the life cycle.

Classification of anaerobic fungi

The ultrastructural uniqueness of the anaerobic fungi, their adaptation to the digestive tract of herbivores and their distribution throughout phylogenetically diverse animals implies that they could have existed as a separate group since the time these mammals began to diverge at least 120 million years ago. Although comparatively little is known about the taxonomy of anaerobic fungi, it is generally agreed that they are zoospore-producing fungi and should be assigned to the class Chytridiomycetes. The order Spizellomycetales in the Chytridiomycetes was established by Barr (2) by subdivision of the Chytridiales to take account of differences in zoospore ultrastructure of the incumbent species. There are, however, many similarities between the families and genera of both orders (the Spizellomycetales and the Chytridiales). At present, anaerobic fungi are classified as follows (4), (5):–

Division	Eumycotina
Sub-division	Mastigomycotina
Class	Chytridiomycetes
Order	Spizellomycetales
Family	Neocallimasticaceae
Genera	Caecomyces, Piromyces,
	Neocallimastix, Anaeromyces
	and Orpinomyces

Recently, Li & Heath (37) and Li *et al.* (38) suggested that the Chytridiales and aerobic Spizellomycetales are more closely related to each other than to anaerobic fungi and that consequently the latter may not belong to the Spizellomycetales. For this reason, they suggested that anaerobic fungi should be assigned to a new order, the Neocallimasticales.

If an evolutionary relationship between anaerobic fungi and aerobic chytrids is to be established and if the classification of the Chytridiomycetes is to be based upon phylogenetic relationships, it is important to obtain information about (a) the GC ratios and (b) the 5S and 18S ribosomal RNA sequences (29) of aerobic and anaerobic Chytridiomycetes. The ribosomal genes of *Neocallimastix* are arranged as tandem repeats with a size of 9.4–10.0 Kb, the average GC content of this region being *ca.* 30% (12). Therefore, although these organisms have different phenotypes (monocentric or polycentric thalli, uniflagellate or polyflagellate zoospores, etc.), it seems that they form a homogenous group with respect to GC content. Analysis of 18S ribosomal RNA sequences has been used to clarify the phylogenetic relationships between the anaerobic fungi, the aerobic chytrids and other eukaryotes. Doré & Stahl (14), Bowman *et al.* (8) and Li & Heath (37) have used partial 18S rRNA sequence analysis to support the assignment of the anaerobic fungi to the Chytridiomycetes, as opposed to the protists, and the inclusion of the Chytridiomycetes with the fungi. It is agreed that anaerobic fungi make up a monophyletic group with 97–99% rRNA sequence similarity (14), although relationships within the group are not yet clear. Analysis of the internal spacer I (ITSI) region of the rRNA gene sequence suggests that *Neocallimastix* (polyflagellate zoospores), *Piromyces* (monoflagellate zoospores) and *Orpinomyces* (polyflagellate zoospores) are closely related whereas *Anaeromyces* (monoflagellate zoospores) is more distant to these genera (37). However, Munn (42) considers that the possession of polyflagellated or monoflagellated zoospores is not a trivial difference and suggests that a family (separate from the Neocallimasticaceae which would continue to contain polyflagellate anaerobic fungi) should be erected to accommodate the monoflagellated species of anaerobic fungi. Sequence data alone cannot solve all the taxonomic questions raised by the anaerobic fungi: for example there is a need to compare the results of different tree-generating algorithms because there is a significant difference of opinion on which gives the most accurate results (19). Cladistic analysis of sequence data, morphological, ultrastructural and other related characteristics will in the future lead to a better understanding of the taxonomic status of these unique micro-organisms.

Table 7.1 SPECIFIC NAMES OF ANAEROBIC FUNGI ISOLATED FROM HERBIVORES

Genus : Characteristics	*Species*	*Source of isolate*	*Ref*
Caecomyces: **Monocentric or polycentric; uniflagellate zoospores; spherical holdfasts**	*Caecomyces communis**	sheep	(18)
	Caecomyces equi	horse	(18)
Piromyces: **Monocentric; uniflagellate zoospores; filamentous rhizomycelium**	*Piromyces communis†*	sheep	(18)
	Piromyces dumbonica	elephant	(36)
	Piromyces mae	horse	(36)
	Piromyces minutis	deer	(27)
	Piromyces rhizinflata	Saharan ass	(11)
	Piromyces spiralis	goat	(28)
Neocallimastix: **Monocentric; polyflagellate zoospores; extensive, filamentous rhizomycelium**	*Neocallimastix frontalis*	sheep	(20)
	Neocallimastix patriciarum‡	sheep	(50)
	Neocallimastix hurleyensis	sheep	(61)
	Neocallimastix variabilis	cow	(25)
Anaeromyces: **Polycentric; uniflagellate zoospores; filamentous rhizomycelium**	*Anaeromyces elegans¶*	cow	(26)
	Anaeromyces mucronatus	sheep	(10)
Orpinomyces: **Polycentric; polyflagellate zoospores; filamentous rhizomycelium**	*Orpinomyces joyonii§*	sheep	(9)

Originally called: **Sphaeromonas communis* (46); †*Piromonas communis* (47); ‡*Neocallimastix frontalis* (45); ¶*Ruminomyces elegans* (24); §*Orpinomyces bovis* (5) and *Neocallimastix joyonii* (9).

Life cycles

MONOCENTRIC AND POLYCENTRIC LIFE CYCLES

In a monocentric fungus, either the encysted zoospore retains the nucleus and enlarges into a zoosporangium [called endogenous zoosporangial development (31), (5)], or the nucleus migrates out of the zoospore, and the zoosporangium is formed in the germ tube or rhizomycelium [called exogenous zoosporangial development (31), (5)]. In monocentric fungi, both types of development result in the formation of one zoosporangium per thallus and only the zoosporangium contains nuclei. In a polycentric fungus, the nucleus migrates out of the encysted zoospore (exogenous zoosporangial development), undergoes mitosis and several zoosporangia are formed per thallus.

NEOCALLIMASTIX SPP (MONOCENTRIC)

Zoospores of *Neocallimastix spp.* have *ca.* 18 posteriorly directed flagella (40, 46); however, for cytological reasons, the higher figure is likely to be 16 rather than 18. Depending on conditions, zoospores remain motile from between a few minutes to up to two hours after liberation from the zoosporangium (40) but, eventually, they are attracted to a suitable substrate (typically a plant fragment) by chemotaxis (48), attach to it, shed or absorb their flagella (43), (40), (20) and encyst. The most remarkable fact about the loss of flagella from encysting zoospores is that there is also loss of kinetosomes and the perikinetosomal apparatus (21). The implications of this are two-fold; firstly, it implies that kinetosomes are not autonomous but arise *de novo* during zoosporogenesis, and secondly, it implies that a mechanism must exist for a rapid fusion of plasma membrane around the site of each deleted kinetosome (42).

Neocallimastix hurleyensis exhibits endogenous zoosporangial development, but *N. variabilis* exhibits both endogenous and exogenous zoosporangium development (25). Lowe *et al.* (40) showed that, during the first 6.5 h of growth of a thallus of *N. hurleyensis*, there was rapid development of an extensive, non-septate, non-nucleate, highly branched rhizomycelium; during this period, the main (germination) rhizoid increased in length exponentially with a doubling time of 2.5 h. Between 6.5 to 9.5 h after inoculation, the rate of extension of the main rhizoid declined, and no further extension occurred after 9.5 h. The zoosporangium initially increased in volume at an exponential rate with a doubling time of 1.6 h, but between 14 to 20 h growth of the zoosporangium decelerated and little growth occurred after 20 h. At *ca.* 21 h after encystment, a septum was formed at the base of the zoosporangium and this event was correlated with a cessation of zoosporangial growth and the onset of zoosporogenesis (at 27 h). The formation of the septum presumably prevented cytoplasm and/or nutrients moving from the rhizomycelium to the zoosporangium. During zoosporogenesis, the protoplasm cleaved to produce uninucleate zoospores which were eventually liberated through a pore formed in the zoosporangial wall opposite the main rhizoid. At 39°C, and under conditions for growth which are unrestricted (nutrients present in excess and an absence of growth inhibitors) the life cycle of *N. hurleyensis* lasts 29–31 h and culminates in the release of an average of 88 zoospores per zoosporangium (40). Thus, assuming that nuclear division in the zoosporangium is synchronous (16), most thalli form 64 or 128 zoospores per zoosporangium. Inoculum concentration has an appreciable effect on the final size of zoosporangia of *N. hurleyensis* (59), and hence on the number of zoospores produced per zoosporangium.

PIROMYCES SPP (MONOCENTRIC)

Zoospores of *Piromyces spp.* have a single posteriorly directed flagellum. Zoosporangium development is either endogenous or exogenous. In the latter case, germination of the zoospore cyst is two sided; initially, a germ tube develops into an extensive, filamentous rhizomycelium as in *Neocallimastix*, but then a tubular outgrowth develops on the side opposite the main rhizoid into which the nucleus migrates to form a zoosporangium at its tip (5). Thus, zoosporangial development is exogenous.

CAECOMYCES SPP (MONOCENTRIC OR POLYCENTRIC)

Caecomyces spp produce zoospores which each have a single posterior flagellum. Upon germination, a cyst of *C. equi* forms a broad germ tube which, unlike *N. hurleyensis* does not branch but instead enlarges into a holdfast (31) which is highly vacuolate and adheres to the substrate (16); this structure has also been called a spherical body (39) vesicle (16) and vegetative cell (62). Development of *C. equi*, like *N. hurleyensis*, is endogenous i.e. the encysted zoospore retains the nucleus and enlarges into a zoosporangium. Consequently, at maturity, the thallus consists of a multinucleate zoosporangium and an anucleate spherical holdfast. For *C. communis*, Orpin (46) observed 'only vegetative structure bearing a *single* sporangium in samples taken from the rumen', but thalli bearing two to three zoosporangia were observed in axenic culture. Similarly, although Wubah & Fuller (62) found that *in vitro* some zoospores of *C. communis* developed endogenously like *C. equi*, others developed exogenously, i.e. the nucleus migrated out of the zoospore into the holdfast. When the latter event occurred, the holdfast contained nuclei and developed two to four sporangial stalks which, at maturity, were terminated in zoosporangia. It may be significant that this polycentric development has only been observed *in vitro* (46).

FILAMENTOUS POLYCENTRIC ANAEROBIC FUNGI

Upon encystment, the zoospore of filamentous polycentric fungi forms a germination rhizoid into which the nucleus migrates (5), (17); the zoospore then becomes redundant (9). A highly branched rhizomycelium develops, with some of the rhizoids containing nuclei. Zoosporangia are formed on sporangiophores produced by the rhizomycelium either singly or in groups of up to six (5), (24); the sporangiophores develop either intercalary or terminally on the rhizoids (5), (9), (24). When mature, the zoosporangium releases zoospores which have 1–16 flagella (9), (10), (24), *Anaeromyces* spp. producing monoflagellated zoospores, and *Orpinomyces joyonii* producing polyflagellated zoospores (Table 7.1). Barr (3) considered the development of polycentric thalli to be a major step in chytridiomycete evolution, as such thalli produce many zoosporangia and have a capability for vegetative reproduction by fragmentation of the rhizomycelium: thus, unlike monocentric fungi, polycentric fungi have indeterminate life cycles and are not dependent upon the formation of zoospores for their continued survival. An important difference between anaerobic fungi which have endogenous and exogenous zoosporangial development is that, although mitosis proceeds in both groups, nuclear migration only occurs in the latter. Osmani *et al.* (52) identified a 22 kD protein (coded by *nudC*) in *Aspergillus nidulans* which is specifically required for nuclear migration and perhaps anaerobic fungi which display endogenous zoosporangial development lack the genes required for nuclear migration.

POLYCLONAL AND MONOCLONAL ANTIBODIES SPECIFIC FOR CERTAIN STAGES IN THE LIFE CYCLE OF ANAEROBIC FUNGI

Antibodies have been produced which differentiate between various structures present in anaerobic fungi. A polyclonal antiserum (SR1 zoo) has been raised in a Balb/c mouse using fixed zoospores from a *Neocallimastix* sp. strain (SR1) isolated from a sheep. This polyclonal antibody recognises a flagellar antigen present along the whole length of the flagellum, corresponding to a 45 Kd protein by western blotting. The antiserum stains all the flagella of a particular SR1 zoospore or none at all. No cross reaction has been observed with any other rumen fungi tested. The strain has been sub-cultured from a single colony to ensure that it is a single clone and the staining pattern on this clone remained the same, suggesting that the appearance or disappearance of the antigen(s) recognised by the antibody may be developmentally regulated.

Injections of washed fungal biomass have also been used to immunise rats for monoclonal and polyclonal antibody production. Three rats injected with strains ED2, SR1 (two *Neocallimastix* strains isolated from sheep) and *Neocallimastix hurleyensis* respectively have produced polyclonal antibodies which recognise most morphological structures including the rhizomycelium, zoosporangia, zoospores and flagella. A monoclonal antibody (CYST 1) has been produced using a rat immunised with strain ED2: immune rat spleen cells were fused with a rat myeloma cell line (Y3AG 1.2.3 (668). The monoclonal produced only recognises an antigen associated with encysted zoospores. Another monoclonal antibody (6DI) raised against *N. hurleyensis* in rat recognizes a surface antigen present on the rhizomycelium but not on zoosporangia or encysted zoospores; this monoclonal cross reacts with crab shell chitin. More recently, fusion involving a rat immunised with *Neocallimastix hurleyensis* has yielded a series of positives and subsequently four cell lines have been cloned. These four positives produced four separate staining patterns in immunofluorescence recognising (a) rhizomycelium, (b) zoosporangia, (c) encysted zoospores, and, (d) flagella, mycelium and zoospores.

Our intention is to use this panel of antibody probes to determine genus-, species- or isolate-specificity and inter-group relationships. They should also be useful in studies of the developmental biology of these organisms and in detection, identification and quantification of specific rumen fungi *in vivo*, i.e. in the rumen.

Gas production as an indicator of the growth of anaerobic fungi

Gas production [as measured by a pressure transducer (58)] has been used to follow the growth of anaerobic fungi in batch culture (Fig. 7.2). *N. hurleyensis* grows exponentially in batch culture with the biomass data giving a specific growth rate of $0.080\,h^{-1}$ (doubling time of 8.7 h) and the biogas data giving a specific growth rate of $0.074\,h^{-1}$ (doubling time of 9.4 h) (34). During the exponential phase of growth there was a high correlation between gas production and culture dry weight, and both biomass indicators showed that the culture entered stationary phase *ca.* 82 h after inoculation. Thus, gas pressure can be used to measure the specific growth rate and yield of anaerobic fungi in batch culture, but cannot be used to follow autolysis. Gas production is a

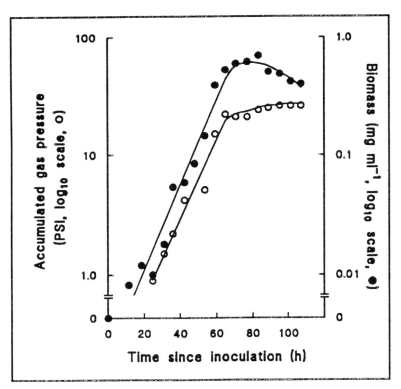

Figure 7.2. Growth of *N. hurleyensis* at 39°C in 100 ml of defined medium B containing 25 mM glucose. The inoculum was taken from 3-day-old cultures grown on the same medium. The gas pressure measurements were made (prior to harvesting the biomass) using a detachable pressure transducer attached to a LED digital readout voltameter. The voltameter was calibrated to read units of pressure in lbs in² [from (34)].

convenient method of following the growth of anaerobic fungi on insoluble substrates such as plant material (35), (57), (34).

Concluding remarks

The generic and specific names of several anaerobic fungi have undergone changes since their fungal status was first recognised (Table 7.1). These changes have created some confusion in the literature and underline the importance of developing molecular mechanisms of classifying and identifying anaerobic fungi.

Acknowledgements

Part of this work was supported by (a) BBSRC funded programme Unit 15 *(Regulation, control and manipulation of rumen function with special reference to rumen microbiology)*, and (b) a research studentship from the *Natural Environment Research Council (Specific detection and enumeration of microbes by a panel of monoclonal antibodies)*.

References

(1) AKIN, D.E., BORNEMAN, W.S. and WINDHAM, W.R. (1988). Rumen fungi: morphological types from Georgia cattle and the attack on forage cell walls. *BioSystems* **21**, 385–391.

(2) BARR, D.J.S. (1980). An outline for the reclassification of the Chytridiales and for a new order the Spizellomycetales. *Canadian Journal of Botany*, **58**, 1171–1201.

(3) BARR, D.J.S. (1983). The zoosporic grouping of plant pathogens. In: *Zoosporic Plant Pathogens*, (Buczacki, T. ed.) pp.161–192. Academic Press Inc. London.

(4) BARR, D.J.S. (1988). How modern systematics relates to the rumen fungi. *BioSystems*, **21**, 351–356.

(5) BARR, D.J.S., KUDO, H., JAKOBER, K.D. and CHENG, K.J. (1989). Morphology and development of rumen fungi: *Neocallimastix* sp. *Piromyces communis* and *Orpinomyces bovis* gen. nov., sp. nov. *Canadian Journal of Botany* **67**, 2815–2824.

(6) BAUCHOP, T. (1979a). Rumen anaerobic fungi of cattle and sheep. *Applied and Environmental Microbiology* **38**, 148–158.

(7)   BAUCHOP, T. (1979b). The rumen anaerobic fungi: colonizers of plant fibre. *Annales de Recherches Veterinaires* **10**, 246–248.

(8)   BOWMAN, B.H., TAYLOR, J.W., BROWNLEE, A.G., LEE, J., LU, S-D. and WHITE, T.J. (1992). Molecular evolution of the fungi: relationship of the Basidiomycetes, Ascomycetes and Chytridiomycetes. *Molecular Biology and Evolution*, **9(2)**, 285–296.

(9)   BRETON, A., BERNALIER, A., BONNEMOY, F., FONTY, G., GAILLARD, B. and GOUET, PH. (1989). Morphological and metabolic characterisation of a new species of strictly anaerobic rumen fungus: *Neocallimastix joyonii*. *FEMS Microbiology Letters* **58**, 309–314.

(10)   BRETON, A., BERNALIER, A., DUSSER, M., FONTY, G., GAILLARD-MARTINIE, B. and GUILLOT, J. (1990). *Anaeromyces mucronatus* nov. gen., nov. sp.. A new strictly anaerobic rumen fungus with polycentric thallus *FEMS Microbiology Letters* **70**, 177–182.

(11)   BRETON, A., DUSSER, M., GAILLARD-MARTINIE, B., GUILLOT, J., MILLET, L. and PRENSIER, G. (1991). *Piromyces rhizinflata* nov. sp., a strictly anaerobic fungus from faeces of the saharan ass; a morphological, metabolic and ultrastructural study. *FEMS Microbiology Letters* **82**, 1–8.

(12)   BROWNLEE, A.G. (1989). A genus-specific, restrictive DNA probe for *Neocallimastix*. In: *The Role of Protozoa and Fungi in Ruminant Digestion* (Nolan, J.V., Leng, R.A. and Demeyer, D.I. eds) pp.251–254. Penambul Books: Australia.

(13)   DAVIES, D.R., THEODOROU, M.K., LAWRENCE, M.I.G. and TRINCI, A.P.J. (1993). Distribution of anaerobic fungi in the digestive tract of cattle and their survival in faeces. *Journal of General Microbiology*, **139**, 1395–1400.

(14)   DORÉ, J. and STAHL, D.A. (1991). Phylogeny of anaerobic rumen Chytridiomycetes inferred from small subunit ribosomal RNA sequence comparison. *Canadian Journal of Botany*, **69**, 1964–1971.

(15)   FONTY, G., GOUET, PH., JOUANY, J-P. and SENAUD, J. (1987). Establishment of the microflora and anaerobic fungi in the rumen of lambs. *Journal of General Microbiology*, **133**, 1835–1843.

(16)   GAILLARD, B. and CITRON, A. (1989). Ultrastructural study

of two rumen fungi: *Piromonas communis* and *Sphaeromonas communis*. *Current Microbiology* **18**, 83–86.

(17) GAILLARD, B., BRETON A. and BERNALIER A. (1989). Study of the nuclear cycle of four species of strictly anaerobic rumen fungi by fluorescence microscopy. *Current Microbiology* **19**, 103–107.

(18) GOLD, J.J., HEATH, I.B. and BAUCHOP, T. (1988). Ultrastructural description of a new chytrid genus of caecum anaerobe, *Caecomyces equi* gen. nov., sp. nov., assigned to the Neocallimasticaceae. *BioSystems* **21**, 403–415.

(19) HASEGAWA, M., KISHINO, H. and SAITOU, N. (1991). On the ML method in molecular phylogenetics. *Journal of Molecular Evolution*, 32, 443–445.

(20) HEATH, I.B., BAUCHOP, T. and SKIPP, R.A. (1983). Assignment of the rumen anaerobe *Neocallimastix frontalis* to the Spizellomycetales (Chytridiomycetes) on the basis of its polyflagellate zoospore ultrastructure. *Canadian Journal of Botany* **61**, 295–307.

(21) HEATH, I.B., KAMINSKY, S.G.W. and BAUCHOP, T. (1986). Basal body loss during fungal zoospore encystment: evidence against centriole autonomy. *Journal of Cell Science* **83**, 135–140.

(22) HO, Y.W., ABDULLAH, N. and JALALUDIN, S. (1988a). Colonization of guinea grass by anaerobic rumen fungi in swamp buffalo and cattle. *Animal Feed Science and Technology* **22**, 161–172.

(23) HO, Y.W., ABDULLAH, N. and JALALUDIN, S. (1988b). Penetrating structures of anaerobic rumen fungi in cattle and swamp buffalo. *Journal of General Microbiology* **134**, 177–181.

(24) HO, Y.W., BAUCHOP, T., ABDULLAH, N. and JALALUDIN, S. (1990). *Ruminomyces elegans* gen. et sp. nov. a polycentric anaerobic rumen fungus from cattle. *Mycotaxon* **38**, 397–405.

(25) HO, Y.W., BARR, D.J.S., ABDULLAH, N., JALALUDIN, S. and KUDO, H. (1993a). *Neocallimastix variabilis*, a new species of anaerobic fungus from the rumen of cattle. *Mycotaxon* **46**, 241–258.

(26) HO, Y.W., BARR, D.J.S., ABDULLAH, N., JALALUDIN, S. and KUDO, H. (1993b). *Anaeromyces*, an earlier name for *Ruminomyces*. *Mycotaxon* **47**, 283–284.

(27) HO, Y.W., BARR, D.J.S., ABDULLAH, N., JALALUDIN, S.

and KUDO, H. (1993c). A new species of *Piromyces* from the rumen of deer in Malaysia. *Mycotaxon* **47**, 285–293.

(28)   HO, Y.W., BARR, D.J.S., ABDULLAH, N., JALALUDIN, S. and KUDO, H. (1993d). *Piromyces spiralis*, a new species of anaerobic fungus from the rumen of goat. *Mycotaxon* **48**, 59–68.

(29)   HORI, H. and OSAWA, S. (1987). Origin and evolution of organisms as deduced from 5S ribosomal RNA sequences. *Molecular Biology and Evolution* **4**, 445.

(30)   HUNGATE, R.E. (1966). *The Rumen and it's Microbes*. Academic Press Inc.: London.

(31)   KARLING, J.S. (1978). *Chytriomycetarum Iconographia: Illustrated and Descriptive Guide to the Chytridiomycetous Genera with a Supplement of the Hyphochytridiomycetes*. J. Cramer, Monticello, NY.

(32)   KOSTYUKOVSKY, V.A., OKUNEV, O.N. and TARAKANOV, B.V. (1991). Description of two anaerobic fungal strains from the bovine rumen and influence of diet on the fungal population *in vivo*. *Journal of General Microbiology* **137**, 1759–1764.

(33)   KUDO, H., JAKOBER, K.D., PHILLIPPE, R.C., CHENG, K.J., BARR, D.J.S. and COSTERTON, J.W. (1990). Isolation and characterisation of cellulolytic anaerobic fungi and associated mycoplasmas from the rumen of a steer fed a roughage diet. *Canadian Journal of Microbiology* **36**, 513–517.

(34)   LAWRENCE, M.I. (1993). *A Study of Anaerobic Fungi Isolated from Ruminants and Monogastric Herbivores*. Ph.D. Thesis, University of Manchester.

(35)   LAWRENCE, M.I., ISAC, D., THEODOROU, M.K. and TRINCI, A.P.J. (1990). Use of head-space gas pressure in batch cultures for determination of wheat straw fermentation by anaerobic fungi. In: *Fourth International Mycological Congress*, (Reisinger, A. and Bresinsky, A. eds.) p. 329. Botanical Institute, University of Regensburg: Regensburg, Germany.

(36)   LI, J., HEATH, I.B. and BAUCHOP, T. (1990). *Piromyces mae* and *Piromyces dumbonica*, two new species of uniflagellate anaerobic chytridiomycete fungi from the hind-gut of the horse and elephant. *Canadian Journal of Botany*, **68**, 1021–1033.

(37)   LI, J. and HEATH, I.B. (1992). The phylogenetic relationships of the anaerobic Chytridiomycetous gut fungi (Neocallimasticaceae) and the Chytridiomycota I: cladistic analysis of rRNA sequences. *Canadian Journal of Botany*, **70**, 1738–1746.

(38) LI, J., HEATH, I.B. and PACKER, L. (1993). The phylogenetic relationships of the anaerobic Chytridiomycetous gut fungi (Neocallimasticaceae) and the Chytridiomycota II: cladistic analysis of structural data and description of Neocallimasticales ord. nov. *Canadian Journal of Botany*, **71**, 393–407.

(39) LOWE, S.E., THEODOROU, M.K. and TRINCI, A.P.J. (1987a). Isolation of anaerobic fungi from saliva and faeces of sheep. *Journal of General Microbiology* **133**, 1829–1834.

(40) LOWE, S.E., GRIFFITH, G.G., MILNE, A., THEODOROU, M.K. and TRINCI, A.P.J. (1987b). Life cycle and growth kinetics of an anaerobic rumen fungus. *Journal of General Microbiology* **133**, 1815–1827.

(41) MILNE, A., THEODOROU, M.K., JORDAN, M.G.C., KING-SPOONER, C. and TRINCI, A.P.J. (1989). Survival of anaerobic fungi in faeces, in saliva, and in pure culture. *Experimental Mycology* **13**, 27–37.

(42) MUNN, E.A. (1994). The ultrastructure of anaerobic fungi. In: *The Anaerobic Fungi* (Orpin, C.G. and Mountfort, D.O. eds). Marcel Dekker: New York. pp 47–105.

(43) MUNN, E.A., ORPIN, C.G. and HALL, F.J. (1981). Ultrastructural studies of the free zoospore of the rumen phycomycete *Neocallimastix frontalis. Journal of General Microbiology* **125**, 311–323.

(44) NOVOZAMSKA, K. (1987). Isolation of an anaerobic cellulolytic fungus from the sheep rumen. *Folia Microbiology* **32(6)**, 519.

(45) ORPIN, C.G. (1975). Studies on the rumen flagellate *Neocallimastix frontalis. Journal of General Microbiology* **91**, 249–262.

(46) ORPIN, C.G. (1976). Studies on the rumen flagellate *Sphaeromonas communis. Journal of General Microbiology* **94**, 270–280.

(47) ORPIN, C.G. (1977). The rumen flagellate *Piromonas communis*: its life-history and invasion of plant material in the rumen. *Journal of General Microbiology* **99**, 107–117.

(48) ORPIN, C.G. and BOUNTIFF, L. (1978). Zoospore chemotaxis in the rumen phycomycete *Neocallimastix frontalis. Journal of General Microbiology* **104**, 113–122.

(49) ORPIN, C.G., MATHIESEN, S.D., GREENWOOD, Y. and BLIX, A. (1985). Seasonal changes in the ruminal microflora of the high-arctic Svalbard reindeer (*Rangifer tarandus platyrhynchus*). *Applied and Environmental Microbiology* **50**, 144–151.

(50) ORPIN, C.G. and MUNN, E.A. (1986). *Neocallimastix patri-*

ciarum sp. nov., a new member of the Neocallimasticaceae inhabiting the rumen of sheep. *Transactions of the British Mycological Society* **86**, 178–181.

(51)   ORPIN, C.G. and JOBLIN, K.N. (1988). The rumen anaerobic fungi. In: *The Rumen Microbial Ecosystem*, (Hobson, P.N. ed.) pp. 129–150. Elsevier Applied Science: London.

(52)   OSMANI, A.H., OSMANI, S.A. and MORRIS, N.R. (1990). The molecular cloning and identification of a gene product specifically required for nuclear movement in *Aspergillus nidulans. The Journal of Cell Biology*, **111**, 543–551.

(53)   PHILLIPS, M.W. (1989). Unusual rumen fungi isolated from northern Australian cattle and water buffalo. In: *The Role of Protozoa and Fungi in Ruminant Digestion* (OECD/UNE International seminar) (Nolan, J.V., Leng, R.A. and Demeyer, D.I. eds.) pp. 247–250. Penambul Books: Armidale, New South Wales, Australia.

(54)   TEUNISSEN, M.J., OPDEN CAMP, H.J.M., ORPIN, C.G., HUIS, J.H.J. and VOGELS, G.D. (1991). Comparison of growth characteristics of anaerobic fungi isolated from ruminant and non-ruminant herbivores during cultivation in a novel defined medium. *Journal of General Microbiology* **137**, 1401–1408.

(55)   THEODOROU, M.K. and KING-SPOONER, C. (1989). Presence or absence of anaerobic fungi in landfill refuse. *Proceedings of Landfill Microbiology Research and Development Workshop*. Energy Technology Support Unit. Department of Energy Publications, U.K.

(56)   THEODOROU, M.K., GILL, M., KING-SPOONER, C. and BEEVER, D.E. (1990). Enumeration of anaerobic chytridiomycetes as thallus forming units: a novel method for the quantification of fibrolytic fungal populations from the digestive tract ecosystem. *Applied and Environmental Microbiology* **56**, 1073–1078.

(57)   THEODOROU, M.K., MERRY, R.J., NIELSEN, B.B., ISAC, D., DAVIES, D.D., LAWRENCE, M. and TRINCI, A.P.J. (1992). A new method for studying growth and activity of surface colonizing micro-organisms. In: *Sixth International Symposium on Microbial Ecology* (ISME–6), Barcelona, 6–11 September 1992. C2–5 Microbial Surface Colonization, p.39.

(58)   THEODOROU, M.K., WILLIAMS, B.A., DHANOA, M.S., MCALLAN, A.B. and FRANCE, J. (1994). A new gas produc-

tion method using a pressure transducer to determine the fermentation kinetics of ruminant feeds. *Animal Feed Science and Technology*, 48, 185–197.

(59) TRINCI, A.P.J., DAVIES, D.R., GULL, K., LAWRENCE, M. NIELSEN, B.B., RICKERS, A. and THEODOROU, M.K. (1994). Anaerobic fungi in herbivorous animals. *Mycological Research*, 98, 129–152.

(60) USHIDA, K. TANUKA, H. and KOJIMA, Y. (1989). A simple *in situ* method for estimating fungal population size in the rumen. *Letters in Applied Microbiology* 9, 109–111.

(61) WEBB, J. and THEODOROU, M.K. (1991). *Neocallimastix hurleyensis* sp. nov., an anaerobic fungi from the ovine rumen. *Canadian Journal of Botany*, **69**, 1220–1224.

(62) WUBAH, D.A. and FULLER, M.S. (1991). Studies on *Caecomyces communis*: morphology and development. *Mycologia* **83**, 303–310.

8

PLANT CELL WALL DEGRADATION BY ANAEROBIC FUNGI

G. FONTY[1,2] and PH. GOUET[1]
*[1]Laboratoire de Microbiologie, INRA, Centre de Recherches de Cler-
mont-Ferrand-Theix, 63122 Saint-Genès-Champanelle, France*
*[2]Laboratoire de Biologie Comparée des Protistes, CNRS, URA 0138,
Université Blaise Pascal, 63170 Aubière, France*

Summary

Anaerobic chytridiomycete fungi that inhabit the gastrointestinal tract
of herbivores, especially the rumen are able to degrade and utilize plant
storage and structural polysaccharides by producing a wide range of
polysaccharide depolymerase and glycoside hydrolase enzymes.
Axenic cultures of fungi are capable of solubilizing a high proportion
of dry weight of even the most highly lignified plant fragments. The
efficiency of these fungi varies according to the species and strains, but
in general, filamentous rhizoïdal species appear better at degrading
plant cell wall than non-filamentous rhizoïdal species. In addition to
their hydrolytic enzyme activity, fungi are able to physically disrupt
plant fibre and weaken the tensile strength of plant material. *In vitro*,
the chytrids have been shown to interact with both fibrolytic and
non-fibrolytic rumen bacteria notably with methanogens.

In vivo, the relative contribution of the fungi to the primary degradation of plant fibre has been the subject of few investigations. In the
developing rumen ecosystem of gnotobiotically reared lambs the efficiency of fungi in plant cell wall breakdown appeared lower than that
of the major cellulolytic bacterial species.

Introduction

The physiological, enzymatic and metabolic properties of anaerobic
Chytridiomycete fungi indicate that these microorganisms might play
an important role not only in ruminal digestion but also in the digestive

ecosystems of non-ruminant herbivores. They have indeed been found in many herbivorous animal species (bovines, ovines, caprines, cervidae, equidae, etc ...) (14, 17, 35, 41). They are present in the lamb rumen from the end of the first week following the animal's birth (19). In adult ruminants, the higher the fibre content of the feed, the higher the fungal population. Diets based on alfalfa or natural meadow hay are particularly favourable to them. On the other hand, starch- rich or soluble sugar- rich diets are unfavourable to them (4, 24, 25). Their ability to colonize plant fragments as soon as they arrive in the rumen, as shown by electron microscopy, their strong cellulolytic and hemicellulolytic activities observed *in vitro*, lead to the belief that they play an active role in the *in vivo* degradation of plant cell walls. This paper concerns the ability of these chytridiomycetes to degrade plant polymers and lignocellulosic tissues *in vitro*, in axenic cultures or in associations with the other rumen microorganisms involved in the trophic chain responsible for the transformation of plant polysaccharides into the end products of fermentation and on the strategy developed by these fungi to digest plant cell wall *in vitro*.

Polysaccharide and sugar utilization, plant cell wall degradation by anaerobic fungi *in vitro*

AXENIC CULTURES

Polysaccharide and sugar utilization

Rumen chytrids use structural polysaccharides and a large variety of soluble sugars for their growth, by producing a wide range of depolymerase and glycoside hydrolase enzymes (17, 18, 21, 27, 35). With the exception of some strains of *Caecomyces communis*, chytridiomycetes are both cellulolytic and xylanolytic. Pectin and polygalacturonate are not, in contrast, generally hydrolysed by fungi. However, a slight growth of polycentric species was observed in culture where pectin was the sole energy source, by Fonty and Bernalier (unpublished results) and a low level of pectinolytic activity was revealed in certain rare strains of *Neocallimastix* (22).

Fungi are able to hydrolyze different types of cellulose, including highly crystalline cellulose. Cellulose degradation requires the adhesion of the fungi to their substrate (13). Indeed, in the presence of methylcellulose, which inhibits fungal adhesion to cellulose, the latter

Table 8.1 FILTER PAPER DEGRADATION BY FIVE ANAEROBIC FUNGAL SPECIES

Fungal cultures	Percentage of dry matter disappearance[1] after:	
	4 days	8 days
Neocallimastix frontalis MCH3	43	78
Piromyces communis FL	60	82
Orpinomyces joyonii NJ1	42	76
Anaeromyces mucronatus BF2	18	60
Caecomyces communis FG10	10	22

[1]100 mg of filter paper were initially placed in incubation.

is no longer degraded. Their efficiency varies according to the species and strain. Strains belonging to the genus *Caecomyces* generally have a far lower level of cellulolytic activity than those belonging to other genera (Table 8.1). The majority of *Neocallimastix frontalis*, *Piromyces communis* and *Orpinomyces joyonii* strains degrade cellulose with greater efficiency than that of the major rumen cellulolytic bacterial species *Fibrobacter succinogenes* and *Ruminococcus flavefaciens* (6, 7). The utilization profile of soluble sugars varies also according to the species and strain (18, 21).

Carbohydrates are fermented by anaerobic fungi via a mixed acid type fermentation, and all fungal isolates examined so far have similar profiles of end products. However, ethanol and formate were not produced by *N. patriciarum* (36) and succinate has been found to be produced by some fungal strains (17).

Plant cell wall degradation

Axenic cultures of fungi are able to solubilize a high proportion of the dry weight of even the most highly lignified plant fragments (31). A mixed fungal population can degrade up to 60% of plant material placed in incubation (3). *Neocallimastix* sp. and *Piromyces* sp. appear to be better than *Caecomyces* sp. at degrading resistant plant tissues. In the case of softer plant tissues, the difference is not so marked (38, 39) (Table 8.2). The efficiency of filamentous rhizoidal species is comparable to that of the rumen cellulolytic bacteria *F. succinogenes* and *R. flavefaciens*.

From a qualitative point of view, observations made under electron microscopy of the degradation of maize or straw fragments by pure

Table 8.2   DEGRADATION OF WHEAT STRAW, RYEGRASS HAY AND MAIZE STEM BY FOUR ANAEROBIC RUMEN FUNGAL SPECIES *IN VITRO* AFTER 6 DAYS OF INCUBATION

| | Percentage of dry matter disappearance [1] | | |
Fungal cultures	Wheat straw	Ryegrass	Maize stem
Neocallimastix frontalis MCH3	35.1	30.0	59.8
Piromyces communis FL	26.5	37.5	60.0
Orpinomyces joyonii NJ1	33.5	35.2	58.7
Caecomyces communis FG10	4.8	11.0	58.0

[1]100 mg of substrates were initially placed in incubation (From Ref. 38, 39)

cultures of the main fungal species reveal that non-ligified tissues such as phloem and medulla parenchyma are the most rapidly degraded, even though lignified tissues are preferentially colonized (23, 26, 38, 39). The aspect of straw and maize stalk tissue degradation by pure cultures is similar for all different filamentous rhizoidal fungal species, monocentric or polycentric alike. *C. communis*, a non-filamentous-rhizoidal species, degrades the same tissues are the other species but with reduced rate and efficiency. No great qualitative difference is observed either between the aspect of the degradation of these plant fragments by fungi or by the major cellulolytic bacterial species of the rumen (38, 39).

Even though no lignolytic activity has been discerned in anaerobic fungi, *N. frontalis* is able to solubilize small amounts of lignin from plant cell walls (27, 34), yet there is no proof that lignin is used as a carbon source. This solubilization is due to the action of esterases which hydrolyze acetyl, uronyl or arabinosyl type bonds, existing between lignin and xylan, and release phenolic acids (10, 46). Rumen fungi are not able to ferment simple phenolic acids. Furthermore, fibre degradation is inhibited in the presence of 10mM concentrations of phenolic acids (1). However, this solubilization, even partial, of the lignin, would increase the accessibility of cellulose and hemicellulose, thus facilitating the colonization and attack of plant particles by bacteria which cannot adhere to lignified cell walls.

The removal of structural polysaccharides and of some lignified components from lignified cell walls would also be expected to considerably affect the properties of plant fragments. Growth of fungi on plant fragments contributes to the diminishing of the tissues' tensile strength, as shown experimentally (2). In fungal culture, a reduction in particle size of wheat straw and rye grass was recorded (34) and Joblin (30) noted that rumen fungi of the *Caecomyces* genus physically disrupt plant fibre by expansion of bulbous rhizoids within the plant tissue. These *in vitro* observations suggest that anaerobic fungi in ruminants assist in the physical breakdown of plant particles. The greater ability of fungi over bacteria to weaken recalcitrant plant cell wall may be important to the ruminant for roughage utilization.

The presence, in the rumen, of several fungal species varying in morphology but similar in metabolic abilities, gives rise to a question: 'What is the function of the differing rhizoidal structures?'. The distinct rhizoidal character of each fungal species suggests that each species has a somewhat different role during fibre breakdown. It is possible that certain fungi may be best adapted to degrade certain types of plant fragments, but little information exists as to this aspect of fungal physiology. The morphological difference between, *C. communis* having a bulbous rhizoid and the other species having an extensive rhizoidal system, probably explains why this fungus is less effective than the other fungi in the degradation of resistant plant tissues, since despite their morphological diversity all species appear similar with respect to the nature and characteristics of their enzymes.

Association of anaerobic fungi with other rumen microorganisms

ASSOCIATION WITH CELLULOLYTIC BACTERIA

Because of their ability to colonize lignocellulosic tissues and of their high cellulolytic activity, anaerobic chytridiomycetes may therefore occupy the same ecological niche as cellulolytic bacteria and interact with them in the rumen. In a coculture with *R. flavefaciens* or *R. albus*, the cellulolytic activity of the main fungal species, with the exception of *C. communis* whose activity is low, was inhibited (7, 37). The quantity of cellulose degraded in fungi/*Ruminococcus* cocultures was therefore smaller than that degraded in fungal monocultures (Table 8.3). This inhibition was due to the release of several polypeptides by the bacteria (8, 40). This inhibition was observed on filter paper and also with natural substrates such as straw and maize (38, 39). These proteins would either act as inhibitors or limit the adhesion of the fungi to the cellulose. It is not known if this inhibition exists *in vivo* in a complex environment and in the presence of numerous proteolytic bacteria. In contrast, fungal cellulolytic activity was not affected in the presence of *F. succinogenes* (8, 38, 39).

Table 8.3　FILTER PAPER DEGRADATION BY THE RUMEN
FUNGI *NEOCALLIMASTIX FRONTALIS* MCH3 AND
PIROMYCES COMMUNIS FL ALONE OR IN ASSOCIATION
WITH *RUMINOCOCCUS FLAVEFACIENS* 007 AFTER 8 DAYS OF
INCUBATION

Microbial cultures	Percentage of dry matter disappearance[1]
N. frontalis MCH3	70
N. frontalis MCH3 + R. flavefaciens 007	42
P. communis FL	78
P. communis FL + R. flavefaciens 007	58

[1]100 mg of filter paper were initially placed in incubation (From Reference 7)

ASSOCIATION WITH H$_2$-UTILIZING BACTERIA

The presence of methanogenic or non-methanogenic hydrogeno-trophic bacteria such as *Selenomonas ruminantium* in fungal cultures led to an acceleration in the rate of cellulolysis, an increase in the amount of degraded cellulose and also in a shift of fungal metabolism towards increased production of acetate, to the detriment of reduced compounds such as ethanol and lactate (5, 32, 33). Thus, estimates of plant cell wall digestion by rumen fungi cultured *in vitro* in pure cultures may underestimate the ability of the fungi to digest the same tissues in the complex ecosystem existing in the rumen. In the presence of *Eubacterium limosum*, a shift of the fungal metabolism was also observed, but fungal cellulolytic activity remained unchanged (9). In the ruminal ecosystem, in the presence of hydrogenotrophic species, fungi will therefore mainly produce acetate and CO$_2$.

ASSOCIATION WITH LACTATE-UTILIZING BACTERIA

Rumen fungi were cocultured with lactate-utilizers from three different bacterial genera. The effects on polysaccharide utilization were, however, inconsistent (40). The rate of cellulose breakdown by *N. frontalis* RE1 was decreased by *S. ruminantium lactylitica*, strain JW13 and *S. ruminantium* subsp. *ruminantrium* JW2. The cellulolytic activity of *P. communis* FL and *N. frontalis* MCH3 was likewise diminished in the presence of *S. ruminantium* strain WLP. Some strains of *S. ruminantium* were also shown to enhance cellulolysis by *N. frontalis* PNK2. Fungal utilization of xylan was also increased by cocultivation with *S.*

ruminantium. Megasphaera elsdenii strain J1/M enhanced filter paper solubilization by *N. frontalis* PNK2. However Bernalier, Masset, Kmet and Fonty (unpublished results) noted a marked decrease in filter paper degradation by *N. fontalis* MCH3, *P. communis* FL, *S. communis* and *Orpinomyces joyonii* when these fungi were cocultured with *M. elsdenii* strain DSM202460. There were also differences between strains in the effect of *Veillonella* species (44).

ASSOCIATION WITH SACCHAROLYTIC BACTERIA

In coculture with *Succinivibrio dextrinosolvens* a saccharolytic species hemicellulose breakdown by *N. frontalis* PNK2 over a 48 hour incubation period was increased from 35% to approximately 75%. In contrast xylan utilization by *N. frontalis* PNK2 was inhibited when cultured in association with non-saccharolytic strains of *Streptococcus bovis* and *Lachnospira multiparus* (45).

ASSOCIATION WITH PROTOZOA

Like fungi, protozoa contribute towards the breakdown of plant fibres in the rumen, there is therefore likely to be a large amount of interaction between both populations during cellulolysis. However, because it is extremely difficult to cultivate ciliates, few studies have been carried out on these interactions.*In vitro*, the presence of *Dasytricha ruminantium* had no effect on cellulose degradation by *N. frontalis.* However, a mixed population of entodiniomorphous ciliates greatly reduced fungal cellulolysis (17, 44). The addition of protozoa to a 48 hour culture of *N. frontalis* in a medium containing xylan, did not effect the degradation of xylan by the fungi over the following 24 hours. Also, simultaneous inoculation and co-incubation of protozoa with *N. frontalis* over a 24 hour period had no effect at all on fungal xylanolytic activity . However, dry matter loss from *Lolium perenne* straw incubated in the presence of *P. communis* was reduced upon the addition of protozoa extracts (44, 45).

MIXED CULTURES

The introduction of a strain of *Neocallimastix* sp into a rumen simulating fermentation system (RUSITEC) resulted in a 15% increase in wheat straw dry matter loss. The breakdown of ADF (acid detergent fiber) and that of NDF (neutral detergent fiber) increased respectively from 15–30% and from 20–30% in the presence of fungi (28).

In vivo plant tissue colonization and degradation

CONVENTIONAL ANIMALS

In the rumen, fungi are attached to plant fragments. Feed particles arriving in the rumen are free of anaerobic fungal spores. Soluble components released by fodder plants induce sporogenesis from the mature sporocytes attached to the plant fragments already present. Thus, it was observed that the number of zoospores increases after feeding. The zoospores, thus generated, are attracted by chemotactism onto the newly ingested fragments and especially onto tissue damaged by mastication (34). With leaves, zoospores can also penetrate through the stomata. This phenomenon, which does not appear to occur with the bacteria and protozoa, allows the fungi to penetrate the cuticle (46). The spores adhere within 15 minutes following the introduction of plant fragments and germinate, thus forming a mycelium that can be observed 3 hours after adhesion (4). The rhizoids penetrate the plant tissue to a depth that can reach up to 460 microns (4, 29) allowing the fungi rapid access to fermentable sugars that are not immediately available to bacteria (29), thus providing them with a significant competitive advantage. Stalks are more abundantly colonized by zoospores than leaves, unless the latter are highly indigestible as is the case in straw. Fungi also preferentially colonize lignified tissues : sclerenchyma, xylem, vascular bundles i.e., those remaining the longest in the rumen (23).

To this day, the specific factors responsible for the development of fungi on different tissues remain unknown and would deserve clarification. In the same way, the modifications in physical structure of plant fragments when under the effect of fungal attack and colonization should be studied in order to better define the mechanical role of fungi *in vivo* in the breakdown of lignocellulosic components. Calderon-Cortes *et al.* (12) indeed observed that the distribution of the size of feed particles in the digesta leaving the rumen was different in the presence or absence of fungi. Quantitatively, the contribution of fungi to *in vivo* cellulolysis and, *a fortiori*, to all the digestive processes in adult ruminants, remains unknown through lack of precise and rigorous means of evaluating it. Their elimination from the sheep rumen after ingestion, by the animal, of chemically treated barley straw, was followed by a sharp decrease in *in sacco* digestibility of straw dry matter (44% of DM loss versus 56% after 48 h of incubation), whereas *in vivo* digestibility remained unchanged (12). However, a question mark can be placed as to these differences resulting purely from the elimination of the fungi, as the chemical treatment of the straw could also have brought about a modification in the microbial populations.

In vivo, the size of the fungal populations and, consequently, their contribution to digestive processes, is affected by the presence of protozoa. Ciliates are often observed on plant material at the adhering sites of sporocytes, which suggests that they can ingest the zoospores when they are released. Although no proof exists of the predation of fungal zoospores by protozoa, it has been shown that the number of zoospores increases in defaunated animals (43, 45). In some cases, however, the number of zoospores remained constant, or only slightly increased, at the time of refaunating. The fungal colonization of straw limbs, estimated by the number of adhering sporocytes, is greater in defaunated animals fed on different straw-based diets, than in faunated animals (45). Electron microscopy studies revealed that certain species of ciliates ingest fungal rhizoids and occasionally sporocytes (17, 43, 45).

GNOTOBIOTIC ANIMALS

The effect of fungi on plant cell wall degradation was assessed, by Fonty *et al.* (16, 20) in the rumen, in various gnotobiotic animal models. Young lambs were placed in sterile isolators 24 h after birth, before the natural establishment of cellulolytic microorganisms and were reared gnotobiotically according to the method described by Fonty and Gouet (16). The lambs were inoculated with fungi as the sole cellulolytic microorganisms and the ability of the established microbial population to digest wheat straw was measured *in sacco*. *N frontalis* MCH3 removed 29.6% and 32.7% of the dry matter from wheat straw after, respectively, 48h and 72h incubation in nylon bags; the cellulose digestibility (Van Soest) was 21.2% and 24.4%. After 48h of incubation the *N. frontalis*-containing population degraded 71% of DM and 36% of cellulose from rye grass hay. The efficiency of *P. communis* FL in degrading these two substrates was similar to that of *N. frontalis* (16). Dry matter and cellulose disappearance were lower in these animals than in conventionally reared lambs and in isolated lambs harbouring *F. succinogenes* S85 or *R. flavefaciens* 007 as the sole cellulolytic microorganisms (16, 17). However, scanning electron microscopy confirmed that the degradation of maize and lucerne stem fragments were similar in animals associated with fungi and in conventionally-reared lambs (16, 17). Interrelationships between fungi and cellulolytic bacteria were also investigated using animal models (20). Interactions between fungi and *R. flavefaciens* were studied in the rumen of lambs isolated 24h after birth. These lambs were then inoculated with pure cultures of *N. frontalis* MCH3 and *P. communis* FL and in a second period with *R. flavefaciens*. Following introduction of the cellulolytic bacterium, there was a significant increase in the disappearance of dry matter and cellulose from ryegrass hay and wheat straw placed in nylon bags. The activity of most of the polysaccharide-degrading enzymes of the microbial populations in the liquid and solid phases, and volatile fatty acid concentration of the rumen also increased.

The establishment of *N. frontalis* in the rumen of lambs isolated 24h after birth and inoculated with *R. flavefaciens* 007 resulted in an increase in straw degradation (34.4% of DM disappearence vs 27.0 after 72h of incubation of the nylon bags in the rumen). In this experiment with meroxenic lambs (20), animals were transferred into sterile isolators 24h after birth, after which they received a 10^{-6} dilution of rumen contents taken from a conventional sheep. A bacterial cellulolytic population was established by this procedure. The animals were subsequently inoculated with pure cultures of *N. frontalis* MCH3 and *P. communis* FL. The presence of fungi in the rumen microbial popu-

Table 8.4   HYDROLYTIC ENZYME ACTIVITIES IN THE MICROBIAL POPULATIONS ASSOCIATED WITH THE DIGESTA SOLIDS OF RUMINAL CONTENTS OF LAMBS RAISED GNOTOBIOTICALLY WITH DEFINED CELLULOLYTIC MICROBIAL POPULATIONS

Enzyme activity	*Cellulolytic bacteria alone*	*Cellulolytic bacteria + fungi*
α-L-arabinofuranosidase	66.2 ± 14.3	143.1 ± 23.8
β-D-xylosidase	25.5 ± 13.7	160.3 ± 11.5
β-D-glucosidase	40.2 ± 19.4	139.1 ± 8.2
β-D-cellobiosidase	15.6 ± 10.4	56.4 ± 11.4
α-D-glucosidase	17.3 ± 14.0	54.7 ± 7.0
Hemicellulase	334 ± 124	931 ± 63.4
Xylanase	242 ± 67.1	668 ± 88.8
Carboxymethylcellulase	162 ± 36.8	464 ± 14.0
Cellulase	64.7 ± 12.5	36.0 ± 17.0

(From Reference 20)

lation had little effect on dry matter disappearence and slightly decreased the VFA concentration, but it increased the activity of most
glucosidases and polysaccharidases of the microbial population adhering to the solid fraction of the rumen contents (Table 8.4).

With gnotobiotic lambs, Fonty *et al.*, (20) also demonstrated that the
synergetic interaction, during cellulose degradation, observed *in vitro*
between anaerobic fungi and H_2-producing cellulolytic bacteria occurs
in vivo.

Conclusions

It is therefore clear, from studies carried out *in vitro* and *in vivo*, that
anaerobic fungi contribute to the degradation of plant cell walls in the
rumen. However, many aspects of their digestive processes as compared to the other biotic elements of the ecosystem, has yet to be
evaluated. In order to do so, it is necessary to know the biomass and the
fluctuations of the fungal population. In the absence of adequate
specific chemical markers and faced with the insufficiency of classic
microbiological techniques, it would appear that only the most modern
tools of microbiology, such as olignucleotide hybridization probes,
might help in solving this problem (11, 15). The inoculation of young
gnotobiotic animals with defined microbial populations offers considerable potential for evaluating the extent and consequences of fungal interactions with the diverse microbial groups that normally reside
within the rumen ecosystem. An important function of the fungi in the
rumen is probably to weaken plant structures, the significance of fungi
in consequence, weakening and physical disruption of plant tissues
must be clarified, in particular by comparing the role of monocentric
and polycentric species having an extensive system of branching fila-
ments with that of *C. communis*, a species that has bulbous rhizoids. In
the same way, the localization of polysaccharidases and glycohydro-
lases along the rhizoidal system, and the metabolic status of the fungal
biomass must also be specified. Indeed, the life cycles of fungi in the
rumen are not synchronised and fungal thalli attached to plant particles will be in various stages of maturation, and little is known about
changes in fungal activities as fungal thalli mature. Lastly, as rumen
bacteria and protozoa interact with fungi and are able to modify fungal
activities, future studies should also focus on the interrelationships
between these three microbial populations.

Increasing our knowledge in the role of anaerobic chytridiomycetes in the breakdown of plant tissues implies numerous further studies whose efficiency depend upon, on the one hand, close collaboration between specialists in ecology, physiology and biochemistry of anaerobes, and on the other hand, the use of modern techniques such as oligonucleotide probes, nuclear magnetic resonance spectroscopy, and image analysis.

References

(1)   AKIN, D.E. and RIGSBY, L.L. (1985). Influence of phenolic acids on rumen fungi. Agronomic Journal, 77, 180–182.
(2)   AKIN, D.E., LYON, C.E., WINDHAM, W.R. and RIGSBY, L.L. (1989). Physical degradation of lignified stem tissues by ruminal fungi. Applied and Environmental Microbiology, 55, 616–616.
(3)   AKIN, D.E., GORDON, G.L.R. and HOGAN, J.P. (1983). Rumen bacterial and fungal degradation of *Digitaria pentzii* grown with or without sulfur. Applied and Environmental Microbiology, 46, 738–748.
(4)   BAUCHOP, T. (1981). The anaerobic fungi in rumen fibre digestion. Agriculture and Environment, 6, 339–348.
(5)   BAUCHOP, T. and MOUNTFORT, D.O. (1981). Cellulose fermentation by a rumen anaerobic fungus in both the absence and the presence of rumen methanogens. Applied and Environmental Microbiology, 42, 1103–1110.
(6)   BERNALIER, A., FONTY, G. and GOUET, Ph. (1991). Cellulose degradation by two rumen anaerobic fungi in monoculture or in coculture with rumen bacteria. Animal Feed Science and Technology, 32, 131–136.
(7)   BERNALIER, A., FONTY, G., BONNEMOY, F. and GOUET, Ph. (1992). Degradation and fermentation of cellulose by the rumen anaerobic fungi in axenic cultures or in association with cellulolytic bacteria. Current Microbiology, 25, 143–148.
(8)   BERNALIER, A., FONTY, G., BONNEMOY, F. and GOUET, Ph. (1993). Inhibition of the cellulolytic activity of *Neocallimastix frontalis* by *Ruminococcus flavefaciens*. Journal of General Microbiology, 139, 873–880.
(9)   BERNALIER, A., FONTY, G., BONNEMOY, F. and GOUET, Ph. (1993). Effect of *Eubacterium limosum*, a ruminal hydrogenotrophic bacterium on the degradation and fermen-

tation of cellulose by three species of rumen anaerobic fungi. Reproduction, Nutrition Dévelopement, 33, 577–584.

(10) BORNEMAN, W.S., HARTLEY, R.D., MORRISON, W.H., AKIN, D.E. and LJUNGDAHL, L.C. (1990). Feruloyl and p-coumaroyl esterases from anaerobic fungi in relation to plant cell wall degradation. Applied Microbiology and Biotechnology, 33, 345–351.

(11) BROWNLEE, A.G. (1989). A genus-specific, repetitive DNA probe for *Neocallimastix*. In 'The Roles of protozoa and fungi in ruminant digestion' (Nolan J.V., Leng R.A., Demeyer D.I., Eds), pp. 251–253. Penambul Books, Armidale, Australia.

(12) CALDERON-CORTES, F.J., ELLIOTT, R. and FORD, C.W. (1989). Influence of rumen fungi on the nutrition of sheep fed forage diets. In 'The role of protozoa and fungi in ruminant digestion' (Nolan J.V., Leng R.A., Demeyer D.I., Eds), pp. 181–187. Penambul Books, Armidale, Australia.

(13) CHENG, K.J., KUDO, H., DUNCAN, S.H. MESBAH, A., STEWART, C.S., BERNALIER A., FONTY, G. and Costerton, J.W. (1991). Prevention of fungal colonization and digestion of cellulose by the addition of methylcellulose. Canadian Journal of Microbiology, 37, 484–487.

(14) CITRON, A., BRETON, A. and FONTY, G. (1987). The rumen anaerobic fungi. Bulletin de l'Institut Pasteur, 85, 329–343.

(15) DORÉ J., BROWNLEE, A., MILLET, L., VIRLOGEUX, I., SAIGNE, M., FONTY, G. and Gouet, Ph. (1993). Ribosomal DNA-targeted hybridization probes for the detection, identification and quantification of anaerobic rumen fungi. Proceedings of the Nutrition Society, 52, 117A.

(16) FONTY, G. and GOUET, Ph. (1989). Establishment of microbial populations in the rumen. Utilization of an animal model to study the role of the different cellulolytic microorganisms *in vivo*. In: The roles of Protozoa and fungi in ruminant digestion (Nolan J.V., Leng R..A., Demeyer D.I., Eds), pp. 39–49. Penambul books, Armidale, Australia.

(17) FONTY, G. and JOBLIN, K.N. (1991). Rumen anaerobic fungi: their role and interactions with other rumen microorganisms in relation to fiber digestion. In : 'Physiological Aspects of Digestion and Metabolism in Ruminants' (Tsuda T., Sasaki Y., Kawashima R., Eds), pp. 655–679. Academic Press, San Diego.

(18) FONTY, G., BERNALIER, A. and GOUET, Ph. (1990). Degradation of lignocellulosic forages by anaerobic rumen

fungi. In 'Advances in Biological Treatment of Lignocellulosic Materials' (Coughlan M.P., Amaral Collaço M.T., Eds) pp. 253–268. Elsevier Applied Science, London and New-York.

(19)   FONTY, G., GOUET, Ph., JOUANY, J.P. and SENAUD, J. (1987). Establishment of the microflora and anaerobic fungi in the rumen of lambs. Journal of General Microbiology, 123, 1835–1843.

(20)   FONTY, G., WILLIAMS, A.G., BONNEMOY, F., MOR-VAN, B., DORÉ J. and GOUET, Ph. (1992). Interactions between cellulolytic bacteria, anaerobic fungi and methanogens in the rumen of gnotobiotic lambs. Proceedings of the International Conference on 'Manipulation of rumen microorganisms to improve efficiency of fermentation and ruminant production'. pp. 338–342. Alexandria, Egypt, 20–23 Sept.

(21)   GORDON, G.L.R. and PHILLIPS, M.W. (1989). Comparative fermentation properties of anaerobic fungi from the rumen. In 'The roles of protozoa and fungi in ruminant digestion' (Nolan J.V., Leng R.A., Demeyer D.I., Eds), pp. 127–128. Penambul books, Armidale, Australia.

(22)   GORDON, G.L.R. and PHILIPS, M.W. (1992). Extracellular pectin lyase produced by *Neocallimastix* sp LM1, a rumen anaerobic fungus. Letters in Applied Microbiology, 15, 113–155.

(23)   GRENET, E. and BARRY, P. (1988). Colonization of thick-walled plant tissues by anaerobic fungi. Animal Feed Science and Technology, 19, 25–31.

(24)   GRENET, E., BRETON, A., BARRY, P. and FONTY, G. (1989). Rumen anaerobic fungi and plant substrates colonization as affected by diet composition. Animal Feed Science and Technology, 26, 55–70.

(25)   GRENET, E., FONTY, G., JAMOT, J. and BONNEMOY, F. (1989). Influence of diet and monensin on development of anaerobic fungi in the rumen, duodenum, caecum and feces of cows. Applied and Environmental Microbiology, 55, 2360–2364.

(26)   GRENET, E., JAMOT, J., FONTY, G. and BERNALIER, A. (1989). Kinetics study of the degradation of wheat straw and maize stem by pure cultures of anaerobic fungi observed by scanning electron microscopy. Asian-Australian Journal of Animal Sciences, 2, 456–457.

(27)   HÉBRAUD, M. and FÈVRE M. (1988). Characterization of glycosides and polysaccharide hydrolases secreted by the rumen anaerobic fungi *Neocallimastix frontalis*, *Sphaeromonas commu-*

nis and *Piromyces communis*. Journal of General Microbiology, 134, 1123–1129.

(28) HILLAIRE, M.C., JOUANY, J.P. and FONTY, G. (1990). Wheat straw degradation in Rusitec, in the presence or absence of rumen anaerobic fungi. Proceeding of the Nutrition Society, 49, 127A.

(29) HO, Y.W., ABDULLAH, N. and JALALUDIN, S. (1988). Penetrating structures of anaerobic rumen fungi in cattle and swamp buffalo. Journal of General Microbiology, 134, 177.

(30) JOBLIN, K.N. (1989). Physical disruption of plant fiber by rumen fungi of the *Sphaeromonas* group. In : 'The roles of protozoa and fungi in ruminant digestion' (Nolan J.V., Leng R.A., Demeyer D.I. Eds), pp. 259–260. Penambul Books, Armidale, Australia.

(31) JOBLIN, K.N. and NAYLOR, G.E. (1989). Fermentation of woods by rumen anaerobic fungi. FEMS Microbiology Letters, 65, 111–122.

(32) JOBLIN, K.N., NAYLOR, G.E. and WILLIAMS, A.G. (1990). The effects of *Methanobrevibacter smithii* on xylanolytic activity of rumen fungi. Applied and Environmental Microbiology, 56, 2287–2295.

(33) MARVIN-SIKKEMA, F.D., RICHARDSON, A.J., STEWART, C.S., GOTTSCHAL, J.C. and PRINS, R.A. (1990). Influence of hydrogen consuming bacteria on cellulose degradation by anaerobic fungi. Applied and Environmental Microbiology, 56, 3793–3797.

(34) ORPIN, C.G., (1983). The role of ciliate protozoa and fungi in the rumen digestion of plant cell walls. Animal Feed Science and Technology, 10, 121–143.

(35) ORPIN, C.G. and JOBLIN, K.N. (1988). The rumen anaerobic fungi. In 'The rumen Microbial Ecosystem' (Hobson P.N., Ed), pp. 129–150. Elsevier Applied Science, London, England.

(36) ORPIN, C.G. and MUNN, E.A. (1986). *Neocallimastix patriciarum* sp. nov, a new member of the *Neocallimasticaceae* inhabiting the rumen of sheep. Transactions of the British Mycological Society, 86, 178–181.

(37) RICHARDSON, A.J., STEWART, C.S., CAMPBELL, G.P., WILSON, A.B. and JOBLIN, K.N. (1986). Influence of coculture with rumen bacteria on the lignocellulolytic activity of phycomycetous fungi from the rumen. Abstract XIV International Congress of Microbiology. PG 2–24, 233.

(38) ROGER, V., BERNALIER, A., GRENET, E., FONTY, G., JAMOT, J. and GOUET, Ph. (1993). Degradation of wheat straw and maize stem by a monocentric and a polycentric rumen fungi, alone or in association with rumen cellulolytic bacteria. Animal Feed Science and Technology, 42, 69–82.

(39) ROGER, V., GRENET, E., JAMOT, J., BERNALIER, A., FONTY, G. and GOUET, Ph. (1992). Degradation of maize stem by two rumen fungal species, *Piromyces communis* and *Caecomyces communis*, in pure cultures or in association with cellulolytic bacteria. Reproduction, Nutrition Dévelopement, 32, 321–329.

(40) STEWART, C.S., DUNCAN, S.H., RICHARDSON, A.J., BLACKWELL, C. and BEGBIE, R. (1992). The inhibition of fungal cellulolysis by cell-free preparation from ruminococci. FEMS Microbiology Letters, 97, 83–88.

(41) TRINCI, A.P.J., LOWE, S.E., MILNE, A. and THEODO-ROU, M.K. (1988). Growth and survival of rumen fungi. Biosystems, 21, 357.

(42) WILLIAMS, A.G. and ORPIN, C.G. (1987). Glycoside hydrolase enzymes present in the zoospore and vegetative growth stages of the rumen fungi *Neocallimastix patriciarum*, *Piromonas communis*, and unidentified isolate, grown on a range of carbohydrates. Canadian Journal of Microbiology, 33, 427–434.

(43) WILLIAMS, A.G. and ORPIN, C.G. (1987). Polysaccharide-degrading enzymes formed by three species of anaerobic rumen fungi on a range of carbohydrate substrates. Canadian Journal of Microbiology, 33, 418–426.

(44) WILLIAMS, A.G., JOBLIN, K.N., BUTLER, R.D., FONTY, G. and BERNALIER, A. (1993). Interactions bactéries-protistes dans le rumen. Année Biologique, XXIII, 13–30.

(45) WILLIAMS, A.G., JOBLIN, K.N. and FONTY, G. (1993). Interactions between the rumen chytrids fungi and other microorganisms. In 'The anaerobic fungi'. pp. 191–227. (Orpin C.G. and Mountfort D.O., Eds). Marcel Dekker, New York.

(46) WUBAH, D.A., AKIN, D.E. and BORNEMAN, W.D. (1993). Biology, fiber degradation and enzymology of anaerobic zoospore fungi. Critical Reviews in Microbiology, 99, 99–115.

9

PRODUCTION OF DEPOLYMERIZING ENZYMES BY ANAEROBIC FUNGI

H.J.M. OP DEN CAMP, R. DIJKERMAN, M.J. TEUNISSEN and C. VAN DER DRIFT
Department of Microbiology & Evolutionary Biology, Faculty of Science, University of Nijmegen, Toernooiveld 1, NL-6525 ED Nijmegen, The Netherlands

Summary

Anaerobic fungi are of biotechnological interest because of their production and secretion of a broad range of polysaccharide-degrading enzymes. Research on these enzymes started about 8 years ago. So far the following enzyme activities have been identified: endoglucanase, exoglucohydrolase, exocellobiohydrolase, β-glucosidase, endoxylanase, β-xylosidase, feruloylesterase, p-coumaroylesterase, β-fucosidase, amylase, pectin lyase and protease. (Hemi)cellulolytic enzymes which have a high specific activity and a low sensitivity to product inhibition are studied most intensively. A review is given of activities and production of these enzymes. The mass cultivation of the anaerobic fungus *Piromyces* E2 in a 10 l fermentor is reported for the first time. (Hemi)cellulolytic enzymes produced in this way have a high specific activity. An application study in which a cellulolytic preparation of *Piromyces* E2 is compared with commercial preparations derived from aerobic fungi is described. The results accentuate the applicability of enzymes from anaerobic fungi.

Introduction

Anaerobic fungi isolated from the digestive tract or faeces of herbivorous mammals, both ruminants and non-ruminants, are of biotechnological interest because of their production and secretion of a broad range of polysaccharide-degrading enzymes. These enzymes provide the fungi with the potential to degrade the major structural compounds in plant cell walls. This paper gives an overview of the depolymerizing activities found so far, and focuses on the production and secretion of (hemi)cellulolytic enzymes. Concerning biotechnological application the cultivation of the anaerobic fungus *Piromyces* strain E2 in semi-continuous culture and in fermentors is discussed. Further, a comparison is made between commercial and *Piromyces* strain E2 enzyme preparations.

Extracellular enzyme activities

Anaerobic fungi grow on a range of structural carbohydrates present in forage fiber. Ultrastructural data on the fiber-degrading capacity of anaerobic fungi were recently reviewed by Wubah *et al.* (43). Rhizoids of vegetative thalli attack cell walls by penetration via stomata and cracks in the epidermal layer. This phenomenon gives anaerobic fungi an advantage over protozoa and bacteria in the degradation of recalcitrant tissues and reduces the textural strength of plant material. Lignin may be solubilized from plant cell walls by depolymerizing enzymes but is not degraded or utilized by anaerobic fungi.

Anaerobic fungi secrete a broad range of enzymes during growth on various soluble (glucose, cellobiose, fructose, xylose, lactose, mannose) and insoluble (several celluloses, xylan, pectin, lucerne, bermuda grass, wheat, starch) carbon sources. The following activities have been reported: endoglucanase (2, 3, 6, 9, 10, 12, 15, 21, 23, 26, 31, 33, 36, 41, 42, 44); exoglucohydrolase (31); exocellobiohydrolase (6, 23, 26, 38, 41, 44); β-glucosidase (11, 19, 20, 22, 31, 33, 34, 36, 39, 42), endoxylanase (6, 20, 29, 31, 33, 35, 36); β-xylosidase (14, 18, 20, 33); feruloylesterase (7, 13); p-coumaroylesterase (7, 8, 13); β-fucosidase (19); amylase (28); pectin lyase (16); protease (1, 24, 40).

Activities of (hemi)cellulolytic enzymes from anaerobic fungi

The degradation of cellulose by aerobic fungi requires the action of at least three different enzymes, an endoglucanase, an exoglucanase and a β-glucosidase (37). The initiation of cellulose degradation (amorphogenesis) by anaerobic fungi most likely takes place by another mechanism than the oxidative or other non-hydrolytic processes described for aerobic fungi. An enzyme preparation from *Neocallimastix frontalis* solubilizes highly crystalline cotton cellulose (39). An exocellobio-

Table 9.1 SUMMARY OF (HEMI)CELLULOLYTIC ENZYME ACTIVITIES
REPORTED

| | | Enzyme activity $(IU.mg^{-1})$* | | |
	Endoglucanase	Exoglucanase	β-Glucosidase	Xylanase
Soluble substrate				
Lactose	2.3–19.8	0.02–0.5	0.8–1.2	47–170
Xylose	2.4–5.4	0.03–0.06	0.1–0.5	25–55
Fructose	2.1–10.2	0.04–0.17	0.2–0.6	28–54
Glucose	2.3–5.8	0.03–0.08	0.3–0.5	28–41
Cellobiose	1.6–6.6	0.06–0.11	0.2–0.5	21–48
Insoluble substrates				
Bagasse	2.2–2.4	0.01–0.04	0.1–0.5	34–57
Wheat bran	1.8–2.8	0.01–0.10	0.1–0.5	13–76
Wheat straw	1.2–4.9	0.01–0.08	0.1–0.9	27–90
Starch	5.7–9.0	0.07–0.16	0.3–1.3	42–122
Bermuda grass	2.0–3.0	0.11–0.20	1.3–2.1	13–20
Cellulose	6.4–21.9	0.10–0.70	0.3–0.7	31–61
Xylan	2.3–7.5	0.08–0.23	0.2–1.0	32–155

*Activities given are composed from values reported in references (2, 3, 6, 9, 10, 11, 12, 15, 21, 23, 26, 29, 31, 33, 34, 35, 36, 39, 41, 42, 44). Substrates in assays: endoglucanase, CMC; exoglucanase, Avicel, Sigmacel, filter paper; β-glucosidase, pNPG; xylanase, various xylans

hydrolase is suggested to be responsible for the initial attack on cellulose. Such an enzyme was not purified yet but the product of the *celD* gene from *Neocallimasix patriciarum* was shown to have this activity (44). In addition to these findings, β-glucosidase inhibition studies showed that 60% and more of the activity of extracellular enzymes from *Neocallimastix* and *Piromyces* species acting on Avicel produced glucose suggesting the major exoglucanase to be an exoglucohydrolase (31). The function of this enzyme in the initiation of cellulose degradation remains to be investigated. Table 9.1 gives an overview of the ranges of activities reported in the literature for (hemi)cellulolytic enzymes of anaerobic fungi grown on different substrates. Enzyme production depends on substrates used, and more or less pronounced differences were found (9, 25). Production of (hemi)cellulolytic enzymes was mostly found to be constitutive, but soluble sugars were less effective inducers of cellulase than cellulose. Catabolite regulation of cellulolysis by glucose, cellobiose and starch was reported for a *Piromyces* species (25). Mountfort & Asher (27) demonstrated repression of endoglucanase production of *Neocallimastix frontalis* by glucose and other soluble sugars. However, cellobiose appeared to be a good inducer. For *Piromyces* strains E2 and R1 good induction was observed with fructose, cellobiose and lactose (33, 36).

The specific enzyme activities reported for anaerobic fungi are gener-

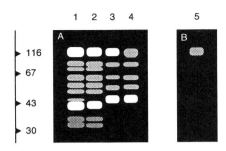

Figure 9.1. β-Glucosidase activity patterns of four anaerobic fungi (A) and β-xylosidase activity pattern of *Neocallimastix* strain N1 (B). Extracellular protein (25 μg) of *Neocallimastix* strains N1 (lane 1 and 5) and N2 (lane 2) and *Piromyces* strains E2 (lane 3) and R1 (lane 4) were separated by SDS-PAGE. SDS-PAGE conditions and activity staining is given in reference (33).

ally high compared to those of members of the aerobic fungal genus *Trichoderma*, which, prior to the discovery of the anaerobic fungi were thought to be the most powerful in hydrolysis of cellulose. The specific activity of CMCases in crude extracellular enzyme preparations from anaerobic fungi is three to six fold higher compared to a hyper-cellulolytic mutant of *Trichoderma reesei* (17) and comparable with a CMCase purified from *Trichoderma viride* (5). Anaerobic fungi can therefore be considered as an attractive alternative for commercial production of depolymerizing enzymes.

The study of the (hemi)cellulolytic enzymes of anaerobic fungi is complicated by the presence of more enzymes with apparently identical functions and the occurrence of High Molecular mass Complexes (HMC, see below) (9, 35, 37, 42). SDS-PAGE with activity staining was described as a method to analyze the presence of different enzymes catalyzing the same reaction (2, 12, 33, 36). An example for β-glucosidase and β-xylosidase activities is given in Fig. 9.1. For β-glucosidase multiple activity bands are present and differences occur between *Piromyces* and *Neocallimastix* strains. For β-xylosidase only one activity band (120 kD) was present which was identical for the strains studied. The SDS-PAGE method was also successfully applied to study the substrate-dependent production of (hemi)cellulolytic enzyme activities (2, 33, 36). Recently we used a preparative isoelectric focusing (IEF) method to study the cellulolytic enzymes of *Piromyces* E2. A typical result of this method is shown in Fig. 9.2. All results obtained demonstrate that the (hemi)cellulolytic enzyme system of anaerobic fungi is diverse and complex. For a complete understanding of the system a detailed study of purified enzymes is needed. So far purification and characterization of β-xylosidases (14, 18), a β-1,4-endo-xylanase (35), β-glucosidases (19, 22, 34) and a p-coumaroylesterase (8) were published.

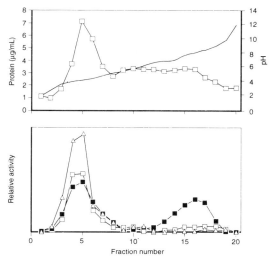

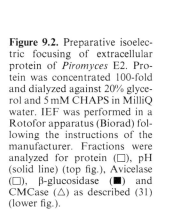

Figure 9.2. Preparative isoelectric focusing of extracellular protein of *Piromyces* E2. Protein was concentrated 100-fold and dialyzed against 20% glycerol and 5 mM CHAPS in MilliQ water. IEF was performed in a Rotofor apparatus (Biorad) following the instructions of the manufacturer. Fractions were analyzed for protein (□), pH (solid line) (top fig.), Avicelase (□), β-glucosidase (■) and CMCase (△) as described (31) (lower fig.).

Production of (hemi)cellulolytic enzymes during growth

PRODUCTION IN BATCH CULTURES

The major fermentation products of anaerobic fungi are formate, acetate, ethanol, lactate, carbon dioxide and hydrogen (37, 43). An example of the degradation of filter paper cellulose during growth on a defined medium by four different strains of anaerobic fungi is shown in Fig. 9.3 (31). After a lag phase (8–48 h) about 90% of the cellulose was degraded within a period of 41 h. The maximum cellulose digestion rates were in the range of 0.13 to 0.25 g.l^{-1}.h^{-1}. These rates are 2 to 7 fold higher than those reported for other *Neocallimastix* strains (4, 23, 30). Digestion of cellulose and production of (hemi)cellulolytic enzyme activities proceeded in a more or less similar way during growth (Fig. 9.3). However, strains differed in the maximum levels of activity. Tsai & Calza (38) performed optimization studies through variations of feeding protocols (fed batch) and inoculation procedures. Remarkable high concentrations of β-glucosidase were found, while other enzyme activities were hardly affected.

PRODUCTION IN SEMI-CONTINUOUS AND FERMENTOR CULTURES

From the point of view of economical production of (hemi)cellulolytic enzymes from anaerobic fungi, it is desirable to study alternatives for

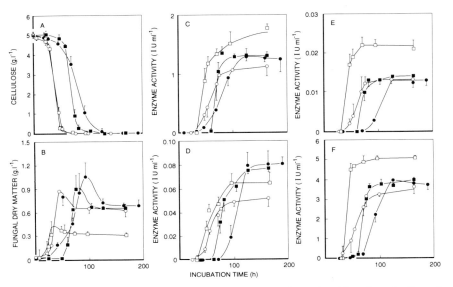

Figure 9.3. Digestion of filter paper cellulose (A), biomass formation (B) and production of CMCase (C), β-glucosidase (D), Avicelase (E) and xylanase (F) by four anaerobic fungi, *Neocallimastix* strains N1 (●) and N2 (■), *Piromyces* strains E2 (□) and R1 (○). Values are means ± S.D. (n=4). Experimental set up is described by Teunissen *et al.* (31).

large scale production. A semi-continuous cultivation system was developed for *Piromyces* E2 (32). The fungus was retained in the system by means of a filter. The extracellular enzymes and fermentation products were continuously removed via this filter. CMCase, Avicelase, β-glucosidase and xylanase activities during growth on Avicel amounted to 3.4, 0.1, 0.5 and 16.4 IU.mg^{-1}, respectively. These values compare rather well with those found in batch cultures (Table 9.1). Optimization of enzyme production was not studied yet.

As a second alternative for large scale cultivation, *Piromyces* E2 was grown on filter paper cellulose in a 10 l fermentor (Fig. 9.4). Growth was followed by measuring formate and extracellular protein production. A lag-phase of about 41 h was followed by a 30 h period of accelerated growth. During the latter phase activities of (hemi)cellulolytic enzymes sharply increased. Growth rates in fermentor cultures were comparable with small scale (0.5 l) batch cultures. Specific activities of CMCase, Avicelase, β-glucosidase and xylanase were 7.5, 0.1, 0.3 and 5.1 IU.mg^{-1}, respectively. Cellulolytic activities fell within the range reported for batch cultures (Table 9.1). Xylanase activity was about 2-fold lower, however this activity is known to be influenced by type and batch of xylan used. Although optimization has not yet been

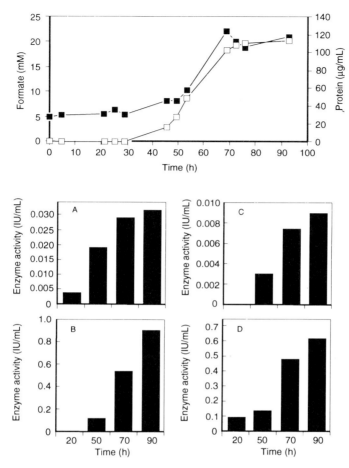

Figure 9.4. Fermentor cultivation of *Piromyces* E2. The fungus was grown on Medium 2 with filter paper cellulose (0.5%, w/v) as carbon source (31). A continuous N_2/CO_2 (80%/20%) gas flow was applied. The fermentor (10 l) was stirred at 180 rpm. Growth was monitored by analysis of formate (■) and secreted protein (□). Activities of β-glucosidase (A), CMCase (B), Avicelase (C) and xylanase (D) are given at four sampling times. Analyses were as described (31).

attempted the results clearly show that large scale cultivation of anaerobic fungi in fermentors with a good production of (hemi)cellulolytic enzymes is possible.

HIGH MOLECULAR MASS COMPLEX

The (hemi)cellulolytic enzymes in cell-free culture filtrates of *N. frontalis* (9, 42) and *Piromyces* E2 (35, 37) are present both in a multicompo-

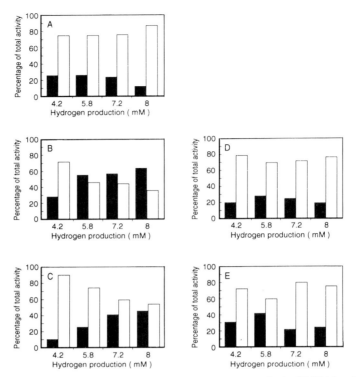

Figure 9.5. Relative amounts of (hemi)cellulolytic enzymes present in the HMC (closed bar) and as free enzymes (open bar) during growth of *Piromyces* E2. The fungus was grown on Medium 2 with filter paper cellulose (0.5%, w/v) (31). H_2 production was used to follow growth. A production of 8 mM indicates the end of growth. Concentrated culture filtrate was applied to a Sephacryl S-300 HR gel permeation column to separate complex-bound and free enzymes. Fractions were analyzed for protein (A), Avicelase (B), CMCase (C), β-glucosidase (D) and xylanase (E) as ddescribed(31). Values are expressed as % of the total activity.

nent High Molecular mass Complex (HMC) and as free enzymes. The molecular masses reported for HMC were 670 kD and 1200 kD. Avicelase activity was almost totally associated with the HMC. The medium composition affected the relative amount of protein associated with the HMC (42). Fig. 9.5 shows the relative amounts of (hemi)cellulolytic enzymes present in the HMC and as free enzymes during growth of *Piromyces* E2. The relative amounts of xylanase and β-glucosidase present in the HMC and as free enzymes did not vary with the growth phase. Both enzymes were mainly present unbound (70 ± 10%). The amount of CMCase and Avicelase present in the HMC increased during growth. At the end of growth about 50 to 60% of both enzymes were complex-bound. Protein distribution appeared to be rather unaffected. Only 25% of the extracellular protein was HMC-bound. At the end of growth even a small increase in free protein was observed.

The physiological function of the HMC in the (hemi)cellulolytic system of anaerobic fungi remains unclear. Concerning this system some analogy with aerobic fungi (synergism) and with bacteria (cellulosome) has been suggested (42).

Application studies

To study the applicability of the (hemi)cellulolytic enzymes of anaerobic fungi a comparison was made with the aerobic fungus *Trichoderma reesei* and commercial preparations (Fig. 9.6). The enzyme preparation of the anaerobic fungus *Piromyces* E2 compares well with the other preparations. Initial activities of Celluclast + Novozym (A) and *Trichoderma reesei* + Novozym (D) were higher but the *Piromyces* enzyme preparations (E, F) retained their activity for a longer period. β-Glucosidase activity of the *Piromyces* enzyme preparations was sufficiently high, addition as with *Trichoderma reesei* was not necessary. This experiment was performed with relatively low concentrations of enzyme. Experiments with higher amounts of enzyme and substrate are in progress. Preliminary experiments revealed that glucose concentrations up to 15 mM did not inhibit the Avicelase activity of *Piromyces*

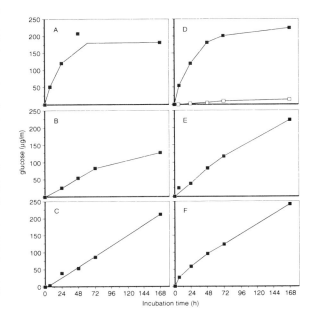

Figure 9.6. Comparison of enzyme preparations from an anaerobic and an aerobic fungus with commercial enzymes. Each incubation contained 5 mg of Avicel in 3.5 ml of buffer (0.1 M acetate pH 5.0 for A-D; 0.1 M phosphate/citrate pH 6.0 for E and F) and 0.5 ml of enzyme solution (all with about 4.10^{-1} IU Avicelase). (A) Celluclast 1.5L + Novozym 188; (B) Maxazyme CL 2000; (C) Celluzyme 0.7 T; (D) *Trichoderma reesei* ATCC 56765, batch culture on Avicel (open symbols), + Novozym 188 (closed symbols); (E) *Piromyces* E2, batch culture on fructose; (F) *Piromyces* E2, semi-continuous culture on Avicel. Formed glucose was analyzed using the GO/POD method (31).

E2. Further, active preparations were obtained after growth of *Piromyces* E2 on agricultural residues (e.g. wheat straw) as substrate.

Perspectives

Anaerobic fungi are identified as producers of (hemi)cellulolytic enzymes with a high specific activity. Further advantages are the absence of product inhibition, the neutral pH (6–7) optima and long term temperature (41°C) stability. Large amounts of enzymes can be obtained by fermentor cultivation. Agricultural residues can be used as a cheap substrate. This will stimulate research on applications. Higher enzyme production can be achieved by isolation of high-producing strains of anaerobic fungi, by genetic manipulation of existing strains and/or by optimization of culture conditions. An alternative approach could be the transformation of genes of (hemi)cellulolytic enzymes of anaerobic fungi into aerobic fungi. Taken into account that research on depolymerizing enzymes of anaerobic fungi only has a short history compared to aerobic fungi major improvements can be expected.

References

(1) ASAO, N., USHIDA, K. and KOJIMA, Y. (1993). Proteolytic activity of rumen fungi belonging to the genera *Neocallimastix* and *Piromyces*. Letters Applied Microbiology 16, 247–250.

(2) BARICHIEVICH, E.M. and CALZA, R.E. (1990a). Supernatant protein and cellulase activities of the anaerobic ruminal fungus *Neocallimastix frontalis* EB 188. Applied Environmental Microbiology 56, 43–48.

(3) BARICHIEVICH, E.M. and CALZA, R.E. (1990b). Media carbon induction of extracellular cellulase activities in *Neocallimastix frontalis* isolate EB188. Current Microbiology 20, 265–271.

(4) BAUCHOP, T. and MOUNTFORT, D.O. (1981). Cellulose fermentation by a rumen anaerobic fungus in both the absence and presence of rumen methanogens. Applied Environmental Microbiology 42, 1103–1110.

(5) BELDMAN, G., SEARLE-VAN LEEUWEN, M.F., ROM-

BOUTS, F.M. and VORAGEN F.G.J. (1985). The cellulases of *Trichoderma viride*. Purification, characterization and comparison of all detectable endoglucanases, exoglucanases and β-glucosidases. European Journal Biochemistry 146, 303–308.

(6)   BORNEMAN, W.S., AKIN, D.E. and LJUNGDAHL, L.G. (1989). Fermentation products and plant cell wall-degrading enzymes produced by monocentric and polycentric anaerobic ruminal fungi. Applied Environmental Microbiology 55, 1066–1073.

(7)   BORNEMAN, W.S., HARTLEY, R.D., MORRISON, W.H., AKIN, D.E. and LJUNGDAHL, L.G. (1990). Feruloyl and p-coumaroyl esterase from anaerobic fungi in relation to plant cell wall degradation. Applied Microbiology Biotechnology 33, 345–351.

(8)   BORNEMAN, W.S., LJUNGDAHL, L.G., HARTLEY, R.D. and AKIN, D.E. (1991). Isolation and characterization of p-coumaroyl esterase from the anaerobic fungus *Neocallimastix* strain MC-2. Applied Environmental Microbiology 57, 2337–2344.

(9)   CALZA, R.E. (1990). Regulation of protein and cellulase excretion in the ruminal fungus *Neocallimastix frontalis* EB 188. Current Microbiology 21, 109–115.

(10)   CALZA, R.E. (1991a). Carbon source, cyclic nucleotide, and protein inhibitor effects on protein and cellulase secretions in *Neocallimastix frontalis* EB 188. Current Microbiology 22, 213–219.

(11)   CALZA, R.E. (1991b). Nascent synthesis and secretion of cellobiase in *Neocallimastix frontalis* EB 188. Current Microbiology 23, 175–180.

(12)   CALZA, R.E. (1991c). Cellulases from *Neocallimastix frontalis* EB188 synthetized in the presence of protein glycosylation inhibitors: measurement of protein molecular weights and isoelectric focusing values. Applied Microbiology Biotechnology 35, 748–752.

(13)   CHRISTOV, L.P. and PRIOR, B.A. (1993) Esterases of xylan-degrading microorganisms: Production, properties, and significance. Enzyme Microbial Technology 15, 460–475.

(14)   GARCIA-CAMPAYO, V. and WOOD, T.M. (1993). Purification and characterization of a β-D-xylosidase from the anaerobic rumen fungus *Neocallimastix frontalis*. Carbohydrate Research 242, 229–245.

(15)   GORDON, G.L.R. and PHILLIPS, M.W. (1989). Degradation and utilization of cellulose and straw by three different anaerobic fungi from the ovine rumen. Applied Environmental Microbiology 55, 1703–1710.

(16)   GORDON, G.L.R. and PHILLIPS, M.W. (1992). Extracellular pectin lyase produced by *Neocallimastix* sp. LM1, a rumen anaerobic fungus. Letters Applied Microbiology 15, 113–115.

(17)   GOSH, A., GOSH, B.K., TRIMINO-VAZQUEZ, H., EVELEIGH, D.E. and MONTENECOURT, B.S. (1984). Cellulase secretion from a hyper-cellulolytic mutant of *Trichoderma reesei* Rut-C30. Archives Microbiology 141, 126–133.

(18)   HEBRAUD, M. and FEVRE, M. (1990a). Purification and characterization of an extracellular β-xylosidase from the rumen anaerobic fungus *Neocallimastix frontalis*. FEMS Microbiology Letters 72, 11–16.

(19)   HEBRAUD, M. and FEVRE, M. (1990b). Purification and characterization of an aspecific glycoside hydrolase from the anaerobic ruminal fungus *Neocallimastix frontalis*. Applied Environmental Microbiology 56, 3164–3169.

(20)   JOBLIN, K.N. and WILLIAMS, A.G. (1991). Effect of cocultivation of ruminal chytrid fungi with *Methanobrevibacter smithii* on lucerne stem degradation and extracellular fungal enzyme activities. Letters Applied Microbiology 12, 121–124.

(21)   LI, X. and CALZA, R.E. (1991a). Cellulases from *Neocallimastix frontalis* EB188 synthesized in the presence of glycosylation inhibitors: measurement of pH and temperature optima, protease and ion sensitivities. Applied Microbiology Biotechnology 35, 741–747.

(22)   LI, X. and CALZA, R.E. (1991b). Purification and characterization of an extracellular β-glucosidase from the rumen fungus *Neocallimastix frontalis* EB 188. Enzyme Microbiology Technology 13, 622–628.

(23)   LOWE, S.E., THEODOROU, M.K. and TRINCI, A.P.J. (1987). Cellulases and xylanase of an anaerobic rumen fungus grown on wheat straw, wheat straw holocellulose, cellulose and xylan. Applied Environmental Microbiology 53, 1216–1223.

(24)   MICHEL, V., FONTY, G., MILLET, L., BONNEMOY, F. and GOUET, P. (1993). In vitro study of the proteolytic activity of rumen anaerobic fungi. FEMS Microbiology Letters 110, 5–10.

(25) MORRISON, M., MACKIE, R.I. and KISTNER, A. (1990). Evidence that cellulolysis by an anaerobic fungus is catabolite regulated by glucose, cellobiose, and soluble starch. Applied Environmental Microbiology 56, 3227–3229.

(26) MOUNTFORT, D.O. (1987). The rumen anaerobic fungi. FEMS Microbiology Reviews 46, 411–419.

(27) MOUNTFORT, D.O. and ASHER, R.A. (1985). Production and regulation of cellulase by two strains of the rumen anaerobic fungus *Neocallimastix frontalis*. Applied Environmental Microbiology 49, 1314–1322.

(28) MOUNTFORT, D.O. and ASHER, R.A. (1988). Production of α-amylase by the ruminal anaerobic fungus *Neocallimastix frontalis.* Applied Environmental Microbiology 54, 2293–2299.

(29) MOUNTFORT, D.O. and ASHER, R.A. (1989). Production of xylanase by the ruminal anaerobic fungus *Neocallimastix frontalis*. Applied Environmental Microbiology 55, 1016–1022.

(30) PHILLIPS, M.W. and GORDON, G.L.R. (1989). Growth characteristics on cellobiose of three different anaerobic fungi isolated from the ovine rumen. Applied Environmental Microbiology 55, 1695–1702.

(31) TEUNISSEN, M.J., SMITS, A.A.M., OP DEN CAMP, H.J.M., HUIS IN 'T VELD, J.H.J. and Vogels, G.D. (1991). Fermentation of cellulose and production of cellulolytic and xylanolytic enzymes by anaerobic fungi from ruminant and non-ruminant herbivores. Archives Microbiology 156, 290–296.

(32) TEUNISSEN, M.J., BAERENDS, R.J.S., KNELISSEN, R.A.G., OP DEN CAMP, H.J.M. and VOGELS, G.D. (1992). A semi-continuous culture system for production of cellulolytic and xylanolytic enzymes by the anaerobic fungus *Piromyces* sp. strain E2. Applied Microbiology Biotechnology 38, 28–33.

(33) TEUNISSEN, M.J., DE KORT, G.V.M., OP DEN CAMP, H.J.M. and HUIS, IN 'T VELD, J.H.J. (1992). Production of cellulolytic and xylanolytic enzymes during growth of the anaerobic fungus *Piromyces* sp. on different substrates. Journal General Microbiology 138, 176–182.

(34) TEUNISSEN, M.J., LAHAYE, D.H.T.P., HUIS IN 'T VELD, J.H.J. and VOGELS, G.D. (1992). Purification and characterization of an extracellular β-glucosidase from the anaerobic fungus *Piromyces* sp. strain E2. Archives Microbiology 158, 276–281.

(35) TEUNISSEN, M.J., HERMANS, J.M.H., HUIS IN 'T VELD, J.H.J. and VOGELS, G.D. (1993). Purification and characterization of a complex bound and a free β-1,4-endoxylanase from the culture fluid of the anaerobic fungus *Piromyces* sp. strain E2. Archives Microbiology 159, 265–271.

(36) TEUNISSEN, M.J., DE KORT, G.V.M., OP DEN CAMP, H.J.M. and VOGELS, G.D. (1993). Production of cellulolytic and xylanolytic enzymes during growth of anaerobic fungi from ruminant and non-ruminant herbivores on different substrates. Applied Biochemistry Biotechnology 39, 177–189.

(37) TEUNISSEN, M.J. and OP DEN CAMP, H.J.M. (1993). Anaerobic fungi and their cellulolytic and xylanolytic enzymes. Antonie van Leeuwenhoek 63, 63–76.

(38) TSAI, K.P. and CALZA, R.E (1993). Optimization of protein and cellulase secretion in *Neocallimastix frontalis* EB188. Applied Microbiology Biotechnology 39, 477–482.

(39) WOOD, T.M., WILSON, C.A., McCRAE, S.I. and JOBLIN, K.N. (1986). A highly active extracellular cellulase from the anaerobic rumen fungus *Neocallimastix frontalis*. FEMS Microbiology Letters 34, 37–41.

(40) WALLACE, R.J. and JOBLIN, K.N. (1985). Proteolytic activity of a rumen anaerobic fungus. FEMS Microbiology Letters 29, 19–25.

(41) WILLIAMS, A.G. and ORPIN, C.G. (1987). Polysaccharide-degrading enzymes formed by three species of anaerobic rumen fungi grown on a range of carbohydrate substrates. Canadian Journal Microbiology 33, 418–426.

(42) WILSON, C.A. and WOOD, T.M. (1992). Studies on the cellulase of the rumen anaerobic fungus *Neocallimastix frontalis*, with special reference to the capacity of the enzyme to degrade crystalline cellulose. Enzyme Microbial Technology 14, 258–264.

(43) WUBAH, D.A., AKIN, D.E. and BORNEMAN, W.S. (1993). Biology, fiber-degradation, and enzymology of anaerobic zoosporic fungi. Critical Reviews Microbiology 19, 99–115.

(44) XUE, G.-P., GOBIUS, K.S. and ORPIN, C.G. (1992). A novel polysaccharide hydrolase cDNA (*celD*) from *Neocallimastix patriciarum* encoding three multi-functional catalytic domains with high endoglucanase, cellobiohydrolase and xylanase activities. Journal General Microbiology 138, 1413–1420.

10

THE XYLANOLYTIC SYSTEM OF RUMEN ANAEROBIC FUNGI

B. GOMEZ DE SEGURA, R. DURAND, C. RASCLE, C. FISSEUX and M. FEVRE
Laboratoire de Biologie Cellulaire Fongique. UMR CNRS 106, Université Lyon I (Bat 405), 43 bd du 11 Novembre 1918, 69622 Villeurbanne Cedex, France

Summary

Rumen anaerobic fungi produce the same range of enzymes with similar properties able to degrade cellulose and hemicellulose. Among the hemicellulose degrading enzymes, xylanases are of importance by degrading and removing the polymers masking cellulose. Three exocellular xylanases have been purified and their properties studied. Two enzymes characterized as endo-xylanases exhibited also carboxymethylcellulase activity. The third enzyme was an exo-xylanase. Secretion of xylanolytic enzymes followed by analytical IEF and western blot using antibodies against endoxylanase I, demonstrated that part of the lytic system is produced constitutively. Endo-xylanases are mainly exocellular enzymes while the exoxylanase is membrane-bound and cell wall-associated. These differences may reflect the respective roles they play in the production of the xylanolytic system and in the degradation of xylans. Using oligonucleotides derived from consensus sequences of xylanase genes, a fragment has been amplified from genomic DNA and used to clone a xylanase gene. Characterization of this gene and searching for other homologous sequences will allow study of the molecular genetics of this xylanolytic system.

Introduction

Cell walls of forage plants have three major biodegradable polymers: cellulose, hemicellulose and pectin. Pectin and hemicellulose associated to lignin, surround cellulose fibrils and constitute a 'barrier' restricting the cellulolytic hydrolysis (1). To degrade and to utilize plant cell walls, anaerobic fungi produce a range of enzymes which have cellulolytic, xylanolytic and amylolytic activities (2, 3, 4, 5, 6).

The complete degradation of plant cell wall polymers implies the successive hydrolysis and removal of the polysaccharides which protect cellulose. In this respect, hydrolysis of xylans is of importance by unmasking cellulose and by providing components utilizable by the host animal or by other microorganisms. Hemicellulose is the second abundant polysaccharide in plant cell walls accounting for up to 40% of the total carbohydrate fraction. The major hemicellulose component, xylan, is a highly branched polymer in which the xylopyranoside units are substituted with acetyl, arabinosyl and glucuronosyl residues (1). Complete degradation of these complex molecules requires the inter-actions of a number of main-chain and side-chain-cleaving enzyme activities. The main chain enzymes involved are endo β-1,4 xylanases, β-1,4 xylosidases and exo-xylanases. Enzymes cleaving side chains would include α-arabinofuranosidase, α-glucuronidase and esterases.

Determinations of the role and the efficiency of the various com-ponents of the xylanolytic systems are of importance for our under-standing of the xylanolysis process mediated by rumen fungi. However, due to their specific properties, these fungal enzymes may find appli-cation in commercial processes.

Complexity and multiplicity of the lytic system

Rumen fungal isolates have very wide ranging polysaccharidase and glycosidase hydrolase activities which allow them to grow and utilize a variety of homo- and heteropolysacccharides. These fungi possess the glycoside hydrolase activities that complement the polysaccharidase enzymes which are also formed, confering an enzymatic potential to release monosaccharides from each plant cell wall polymer (2, 3) . Comparison of the equipment of different species, *Neocallimastix frontalis, Sphaeromonas communis* and *Piromonas communis* revealed that they exhibited the same range and nature of exo and endo-acting enzymes (Table 10.1). These enzymes were mainly secreted and their activities were of the same magnitude when the fungi were grown in the presence of sisal fibers. The enzymatic properties (optimum pH and temperature, Km) were similar from one enzyme activity to another and from a species to another. From these data, it appears that the different fungal species may fulfil similar roles in the rumen.

Table 10.1 COMPARISON OF THE PROPERTIES OF THE HYDROLASES
SECRETED BY *N. FRONTALIS (N.F.) S. COMMUNIS (S.C.)* and *P. COMMUNIS (P.C.)*

	Optimum temperature °C			Optimum pH			Km (mg substrate ml^{-1})		
	N.f.	*S.c.*	*P.c.*	*N.f.*	*S.c.*	*P.c.*	*N.f.*	*S.c.*	*P.c.*
β-Glucosidase	50	50	50	6.0	6.0	6.0	0.55	0.51	0.52
β-Fucosidase	55	55	55	6.0–6.5	6.0–6.5	6.0–6.5	0.39	0.37	0.30
β-Xylosidase	35	39	39	6.5	6.5	6.0–6.5	0.34	0.36	0.40
β-Galacto-sidase	50	50	50	6.0	6.0	6.0	1.89	1.20	1.24
β-1,3-Glucanase	55	55	55	6.0	6.0	6.0	0.97	0.85	0.77
β-1,4-Glucanase	45	50	50	5.5	5.5	6.0	2.79	2.89	2.43
Xylanase	50	50	50	6.0	6.0	5.5	1.13	0.98	1.00

   The complexity of the lytic system is reinforced by the multiplicity of
the enzymatic forms. Chromatographic analysis and analytical IEFs of
the secreted proteins followed by the revelation of their enzymatic
activity revealed this multiplicity (8, 9). Several proteins migrating at
different pHs or differing in their molecular weights exhibited the same
enzyme activity. For example, 19 xylanase and 11 cellulase activity
bands have been resolved from extracellular proteins secreted by *N.
frontalis* (9). The enzyme multiplicity may confer a greater adaptive
capacity to the fungus to degrade a wide range of plants. However, the
origin of this multiplicity is unknown. A specificity of the enzymes
could be implicated in the apparent multiplicity. Different activities
were exhibited at the same pH indicating the non specific action of an
enzyme on several substrates. For example a glycoside hydrolase from
N. frontalis exhibiting βglucosidase, β-fucosidase and β-galactosidase
activities has been characterized and purified (10). Post-secretional
modifications such as moderate proteolysis could also be involved in
the existence of different molecular forms of the enzymes. If little post
secretional modification occurs, this suggests that the multiplicity is
due to the expression of gene families.

Characterization of xylanolytic enzymes from *N. frontalis*

Exocellular hemicellulolytic enzymes from *N. frontalis* consist of a
mixture of xylanase and xylosidase activities. In order to appreciate
their respective role in fiber digestion, xylanase and xylosidase have
been purified (9, 11, 12). Following anion exchange chromatography

Table 10.2   PROPERTIES OF THE PURIFIED XYLANOLYTIC ENZYMES
PRODUCED BY *N. FRONTALIS* (9, 11, 12) MW CORRESPONDING TO MW
SUBUNITS. MW OF NATIVE FORMS ARE INDICATED IN BRACKETS.

	xylanase 1	*xylanase 2*	*exoxylanase*	*xylosidase*
MW	45	70	90(80)	92–46(140)
T°C	50–55	55	35	–
pH	6	5.5	6–6.5	–
Km	1.22	2.5	0.33	–

and gel filtration chromatography, two endoxylanases, an exoxylanase
and a β-xylosidase were purified to homogeneity (Table 10.2). The
exoenzymes which had a high apparent molecular weight as suggested
by gel filtration were separated into two subunits as revealed by SDS-
PAGE (9–11). On the contrary the endoxylanase activities consisted of
single proteins of a lower molecular weight (12). Similar data have been
obtained with a β-xylosidase from another strain of *N. frontalis* (10)
and with xylanases from *Piromyces* (14).All these purified enzymes
showed optimal activity at pH 5.5 to 6. The optimal temperature was
50–55°C for the endo-enzymes and 35°C for the exo-enzymes. These
enzymes were sensitive to small variations of pH or temperature as
their activities decreased rapidly on both sides of the maximal values
(11–12). The optimum of activity of the enzymes is clearly related to the
physiological conditions of the rumen.

Induction and secretion of xylanolytic enzymes

Production of extracellular xylanase and xylosidase activities as a
function of time in cultures grown on glucose (G), methyl glucoside
(M) xylans (X) or straw (P) as carbon source were monitored (Fig.
10.1). A high xylanase activity was recorded in the methyl glucoside,
straw and xylan cultures. In glucose culture, xylanase activity was 10
times lower. These differences in enzyme activity do not correlate with
the growth yields and show that methyl glucoside, straw and xylan are
good inducers of xylanase activity. When glucose was added to these
inducers, xylanase activity was not induced and corresponded to the
level observed in glucose cultures. The β-xylosidase pattern of production was similar. The enzyme activity induced at different levels in the
presence of xylan, methyl glucoside and straw was repressed in the
presence of glucose.

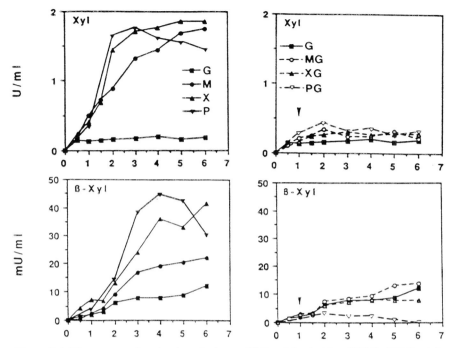

Figure 10.1. Time course of production of xylanase (Xyl) and β xylosidase (β Xyl) of *N. frontalis* grown in the presence of different carbon sources: G, glucose; M, methyl glucoside; X, xylan; P, straw; MG, methyl glucoside and glucose; XG, xylan and glucose; PG, straw and glucose. The arrows indicate the time glucose was added.

Polyclonal antibodies raised against a purified enzyme, endoxylanase I, were used to follow the secretion of the enzyme. Western blots of extracellular proteins revealed the presence of xylanase I in non induced (G), induced (M) and repressed (M + G) cultures indicating the constitutive synthesis of this enzyme (9).The presence of several constitutive xylanase forms was confirmed by analytical IEFs of the proteins secreted into these cultures. The basal activity of the glucose culture corresponded to a limited number of isoforms which were also detected in the repressed cultures. In the induced culture, the high xylanase activity was correlated with the presence of new isoforms. These data indicate that the xylanolytic system from *N. frontalis* is composed by numerous constitutive and regulated isoforms.

Another feature of the xylanolytic system is the different localization of the exo- and endo-enzymes. Different subcellular fractions (cell walls, membranes and soluble fractions) were isolated by differential centrifugation of mycelial extracts and their activities compared to the extracellular fraction (Table 10.3). Xylanase activity was mainly se-

Table 10.3   SUBCELLULAR LOCALIZATION OF XYLANOLYTIC ENZYMES IN *N. FRONTALIS.*

	Xylosidase			*Xylanase*		
	Tot. Act	*Spec. Act*	*%*	*Tot. Act*	*Spec. Act*	*%*
Cytosol	17.4	0.96	33	18.4	1.02	8.2
Membrane	0.9	0.11	2	11.1	1.33	4.9
Cell wall	22.6	0.69	44	16.5	0.5	7.3
Extracellular	10.9	0.38	11	179.2	6.22	79.6

Mycelial cell free extracts were centrifuged at 4000 g for 10 min then at 48 000 g for 30 min to give the cell wall fraction (pellet 4000 g), the membrane fraction (pellet 48 000 g) and the soluble fraction *i.e.* cytosol (supernatant 48 000 g)

creted as about 80 percent of the total activity was recovered in the culture medium. On the contrary xylosidase activity was poorly secreted as only about 10 percent of the total activity was extracellular. This enzyme was mainly associated with the cell wall and the soluble fractions. These differences may reflect the respective roles played by the enzymes in the total degradation and assimilation of xylans. Extracellular xylanases can degrade the polymer into oligosaccharides which will be converted to xylose when entering the cell. Among the enzymes we have purified, xylanases have a lower MW than β xylosidase. One cannot exclude that cell wall porosity could be involved in the sequestration of the β xylosidase.

Molecular cloning of xylanase genes

Sequence alignment and hydrophobic cluster analysis have been utilized to assign polysaccharidases and glycosidases to enzyme families (15). Among these sequences, conserved domains (substrate binding and catalytic domains) have been identified. In order to clone genes encoding xylanase activity, oligonucleotides derived from conserved

a   VEYYIIEDWVDWVPDAQRRMVTIYGFQYKIFQMDHIGPTINGTSETFKQF

b   VEYYIIEDWVDWVPDAQGKMVTIDGAQYKIFQMDHTGPTINGGSETFKQF

a   SVRKQKRTSGHITVSDHFKEWAKQGWGIGNLYEVALNAEGWQSS

b   SVRQQKRTSGHITVSDHFKEWAKQGWGIGNLYEVALNAEGWQSS

Figure 10.2. Comparison of the deduced amino acid sequences of a genomic clone from *N. frontalis* (a) and a cDNA clone from *N. patriciarum* (b) (16) encoding xylanase activity.

sequences were synthesized for PCR amplification of DNA fragments from the genomic DNA of *N. frontalis*. Several fragments were produced using primers corresponding to the catalytic domains of low MW xylanases. Among these fragments one has been sequenced (Fig. 10.2) Comparison with sequences in databases revealed homology between this gene and a cDNA encoding xylanase from *N. patriciarum* and bacterial xylanases. Alignment of homologous regions revealed an identity of 92 percent between the two fungal genes. Using this fragment as a probe, several clones have been isolated from a genomic library and characterized. Comparison of their complete sequences should reveal the extend of homology between genes encoding xylanase activity of the different rumen organisms.

Discussion

Anaerobic fungi have been shown to grow on a range of structural carbohydrates present in forage fiber. They produce cellulolytic and xylanolytic enzymes which possess a high activity. However we don't know if the efficiency is due to specific properties of individual enzymes or to the great number of molecular forms which may have a synergistic and cooperative mode of action.

Biochemical analysis has revealed that the xylanolytic activity is supported by a great number of molecular forms varying in their MW or pI. They may represent different gene products however post translational modifications (glycosylation, proteolysis) may also participate in their multiplicity.

Constitutive levels of xylanase and xylosidase are produced but synthesis of inducible enzymes is promoted by various sugars. Very little work has been done on the regulation of synthesis of the xylanolytic enzymes. Our data showed that xylanases are extracellular proteins of a low MW while β xylosidase are mainly intracellular and of a higher MW. The distribution of the xylanolytic enzymes and their mode of action will thus agree with the generally accepted view on the regulation of enzymes degrading polymeric substrates. Constitutive extracellular xylanases may degrade xylan to xylooligosaccharides which will enter the cell and be degraded by constitutive xylosidase. The degradation products could induce other xylanase and xylosidases genes. However these enzymes are induced by non-related sugars i.e. cellulose, cellobiose (8, 9) and it is possible that identical regulatory mechanisms control xylanase and cellulase synthesis. Molecular genetic studies have to be undertaken to determine structure – function relationships and regulation of individual genes. We have cloned a gene encoding a endoxylanase activity. The homology observed with other rumen organism xylanases raises the problem of possible horizontal transfer of genes between organisms confined in a very specific biotope. Molecular genetics has already revealed particular features of the gene organization of anaerobic fungi compared to aerobic fungal genes (17). Analysis of the xylanase genes, their comparison with prokaryotic and other eukaryotic genes may provide a model to understand the evolution of the anaerobic fungi.

References

(1)   ASPINALL, G.O. (1980). Chemistry of the cell wall polysaccharides. In J. Preiss (ed). The biochemistry of plants. A comprehensive treatise Vol 3. Carbohydrate structure and function. pp 473–500 Academic Press

(2)   WILLIAMS, A.G. and ORPIN, C.G. (1987). Polysaccharide degrading enzymes formed by the three species of anaerobic rumen fungi grown on a range of carbohydrate substrate. Canadian Journal of Microbiology 33, 418–426.

(3)   HEBRAUD, M. and FEVRE, M. (1988). Characterization of glycoside and polysaccharide hydrolases secreted by the rumen anaerobic fungi *Neocallimastix frontalis, Sphaeromonas communis* and *Piromonas communis*. Journal of General Microbiology 134, 1123–1129.

(4)   MOUNTFORT, D.O. and ASHER, R.A. (1985). Production and regulation of cellulase by two strains of the rumen anaerobic fungus *Neocallimastix frontalis*. Applied Environmental Microbiology 49, 1314–1322.

(5)   WOOD, J.M., WILSON, C.A., MACCRAE, S.I. and JOBLIN, N.K. (1986). A highly active extracellular cellulase from the anaerobic fungus *Neocallimastix frontalis*. FEMS Microbiology Letters 34, 37–40.

(6)   LOWE, S.A., THEODOROU, M.K. and TRINCI, A.P.J. (1987). Cellulase and xylanase of an anaerobic rumen fungus grown on wheat straw, wheat, straw holocellulose, cellulose and xylan. Applied Environmental Microbiology 53, 1216–1223.

(7)   TEUNISSEN, M.J. and OP DEN CAMP, H.J.M. (1993). Anaer-

obic fungi and their cellulolytic and xylanolytic enzymes. Antonie van Leeuwenhoeck. 63, 63–76.

(8) HEBRAUD, M. (1988). Production et caractérisation des hydrolases secrétées par les champignons anaérobies du rumen. Thése Université Claude Bernard LYON I.

(9) GOMEZ DE SEGURA, B. (1993). Caractérisation biochimique du système xylanolytique d'un champignon anaérobie du rumen *Neocallimastix frontalis*. Thése Université Claude Bernard LYON I.

(10) HEBRAUD, M. and FEVRE, M. (1990). Purification and characterization of an aspecific glycoside hydrolase from the anaerobic ruminal fungus *Neocallimastix frontalis*. Applied Environmental Microbiology 56, 3164–3169.

(11) HEBRAUD, M. and FEVRE, M. (1990). Purification and characterization of an extracellular β-xylosidase from the rumen anaerobic fungus *Neocallimastix frontalis*. FEMS Microbiology Letters 42, 11–16.

(12) GOMEZ DE SEGURA, B. and FEVRE, M. (1993). Purification and characterization of two 1,4 β xylan endohydrolases from the rumen fungus *Neocallimastix frontalis*. Applied Environmental Microbiology (in the press).

(13) GARCIA CAMPAYO, V. and WOOD, T.M. (1993). Purification and characterization of a β-xylosidase from the anaerobic rumen fungus *Neocallimastix frontalis*. Carbohydrate Research 242, 229–245.

(14) TEUNISSEN, M. (1992). Anaerobic fungi and their cellulolytic and xylanolytic enzymes. Thesis Catholic University of Nijmegen.

(15) GILKES N.R., HENRISSAT B., KILBURN P., MILLER Jr. R.C. and WARREN J.C. (1991). Domains in microbial β 1,4 glycanases: sequence, conservation function and enzyme families. Microbiological Review 55, 303–315.

(16) GILBERT, H.J., HAZLEWOOD, G.P., LAURIE, J.I., ORPIN, C.G. and XUE, G.P. (1992). Homologous catalytic domains in a rumen fungal xylanase: evidence for gene duplication and prokaryotic origin. Molecular Microbiology 6, 2065–2072.

(17) DURAND, R., REYMOND-COTTON, P., FISCHER, M., RASCLE, C. and FEVRE, M. (1993). Cloning and expression of genes encoding enzymes of the glycolytic pathway in *Neocallimastix frontalis*. This volume p 137–151.

11

CLONING AND EXPRESSION OF GENES ENCODING ENZYMES OF THE GLYCOLYTIC PATHWAY IN *NEOCALLIMASTIX FRONTALIS*

R. DURAND, P. REYMOND-COTTON, M. FISCHER,
C. RASCLE and M. FEVRE
*Laboratoire de Biologie Cellulaire Fongique – CGMC UMR CNRS 106,
Université Claude Bernard LYON I (Bat 405), 43 bd 11 Novembre 1918
– 69622 Villeurbanne Cedex – FRANCE*

Summary

The anaerobic fungus *Neocallimastix frontalis* was used as a model to clone the genes encoding enzymes of the glycolytic pathway. Two genes have been isolated from genomic and cDNA libraries : the enolase and phosphoenolpyruvate carboxykinase genes. These genes have been characterized and their sequences compared to the sequences of homologous genes in other organisms. The codon usage observed in the enolase and phosphoenolpyruvate carboxykinase genes is very similar and largely biased as observed in highly expressed fungal genes. The expression of these genes encoding metabolic enzymes studied in cultures grown on different carbon sources demonstrated that the two genes have different transcriptional regulation. Some of the particular features of gene organization in anaerobic fungi are outlined.

Introduction

The anaerobic fungus *Neocallimastix frontalis* can utilize several monosaccharides and plant cell wall polymers as carbon sources (1). The fungus produces a large number of fermentation products from glucose via glycolysis and other metabolic pathways, parts of which are located in microbodies called hydrogenosomes (2).

Neocallimastix frontalis has been intensively studied for its large production of a wide range of glycoside and polysaccharide hydrolases. The production of these enzymes is regulated by the carbon source

137

used for growth. Hydrolase production is induced in the presence of polymers (cellulose, xylans) and repressed in the presence of simple oligocaccharides (3). *Neocallimastix frontalis* was used as a model to clone the genes expressed during hydrolysis of complex plant cell wall polysaccharides and to investigate the molecular mechanisms involved in the regulation of the hydrolase gene expression.

A differential screening of a cDNA library lead to the isolation of several clones which were highly expressed during growth on cellulose (presumably hydrolase genes) and clones which were expressed at high levels during growth on glucose (presumably genes encoding enzymes of metabolic pathways). Several of these clones have been character-ized by restriction endonuclease analysis, sequencing and Northern blotting. Two of these clones have been extensively studied and identi-fied as the enolase gene and the phosphoenolpyruvate carboxykinase gene. The expression of these genes encoding metabolic enzymes has been studied after growing the fungus on different carbon sources.

Cloning and characterization of the *Neocallimastix frontalis* enolase gene (*ENO*)

Preliminary sequence analysis of several cDNA clones isolated by differential screening of a cDNA library showed that a 1.3 kb clone (pPR 61) had an extensive sequence homology with the sequences of the two yeast enolase genes *ENO1* and *ENO 2*. This cDNA clone was characterized by restriction mapping and subcloned. The sequence of overlapping subclones and the deduced amino-acid sequence revealed that the 5' part of the cDNA was missing in the pPR 61 clone. Subsequent screening of two cDNA libraries were unsuccessful for isolating a complete clone.

This partial enolase cDNA clone was used as a probe to screen by plaque hybridization a *N. frontalis* genomic DNA library. A positive clone was characterized by Southern analysis and subcloned. A partial restriction map of the *N. frontalis* insert in plasmid p SKXX67 is shown in Fig. 11.1. Large 5' and 3' flanking non coding regions are present in the clone. The DNA sequence was identified as encoding an enolase on the basis of its high homology to the *Saccharomyces cerevisiae* enolase genes. This is the first characterization and sequencing of an enolase gene from a filamentous fungus while enolase genes have been isolated from the yeasts *Saccharomyces cerevisiae* (4) and *Candida albicans* (5).

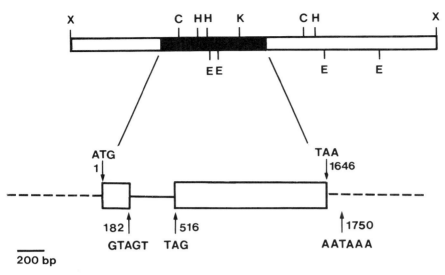

1 kb

200 bp

Figure 11.1. Organization of the *N. frontalis* enolase genomic clone.
Upper part: restriction map of the gene and flanking sequences.
X = Xbal; C = Clal; H = Hind III; E = EcoRI; K = Kpnl
Lower part: structure of the *N. frontalis* *ENO* gene
    Open boxes indicate exons, full line indicates the intron and dashed lines the 5′ and 3′
non-coding sequences. The borders of the intron, the splicing signals and the polyadenylation
consensus sequence are indicated by arrows.

SEQUENCE ANALYSIS

The sequence analysis showed an open reading frame of 1648 bp
interrupted by an intervening sequence of 337 bp (Fig. 11.1). The
protein begins at a typical eukaryotic AUG start codon and terminates
at a UAA stop codon. The 436 amino-acid deduced sequence predicts
for a 47 kD protein.

The G+C content of the coding sequence is 43.8% which is in sharp
contrast to the G+C content of the intervening sequence (14.2%) or the
3′ non-coding sequence (15.2%). Brownlee (6) and Billon *et al.* (7)
pointed out that the overall G+C content of the nuclear DNAs from
several species of anaerobic rumen fungi was very low (less than 20%)
and between 16 to 18% in *Neocallimastix* sp. according to the procedure used. (6,7). These results indicate that the anaerobic fungi have
the most A/T rich genomes of any organism identified so far. The
highly repetitive genes encoding the ribosomal RNA and their flanking

region and the presence of repeated sequences spread in the *N. frontalis* genome could account for the low G+C content of the DNA (6).The very low G+C content of sequences flanking transcribed genes as shown for the enolase clone could also account for the base composition of the DNA of anaerobic fungi. The sequence of the *Neocallimastix frontalis* enolase gene is interrupted by a 337 bp intron (Fig. 11.1). This intron is the largest intron found so far in filamentous fungal genes. Filamentous fungal introns are short, on average less than 100 bp (8). There can be as many as eight intervening sequences in filamentous fungal genes. With regard to location, fungal introns may be situated towards the 5' end or near the 3' end of the gene or randomly distributed throughout the gene. In *S. cerevisiae* the introns present in 10% of the genes have a uniform length of about 300–500 nucleotides and the split genes contain only one intervening sequence located within the extreme 5' part of the primary transcript (9). These features are quite close to the intron size and location observed in *N. frontalis*.

Neocallimastix frontalis ENO intron boundaries are similar to those of yeast, fungi, plants and vertebrates in that they have the nucleotide pair GT and AG bounding their 5' and 3' extremities respectively (8). Comparisons of intron splice junctions in Mastigomycotinae genes are shown in Table 11.1. In *S. cerevisiae*, an intron internal consensus sequence 5'-TACTAAC-3' is known to be necessary for intron splicing. This sequence does not generally appear in fungal introns which exhibit less strict sequence stretches with a general consensus PyGCTAACN(10). The sequence TACTTAAA present in the *N. frontalis ENO* intron showed the CT at positions 4 and 5 of the element and the A at position 6 as they occur in the fungal consensus sequence.

The consensus sequence AAUAAA which is thought to be involved in polyadenylation of the 3' terminus of mature mRNA is present in the 3' part of enolase clone 100 bp downstream to the stop codon. The 3' non coding region showed several repeated inverted sequences forming loops which may be involved in transcription termination (5).

The codon usage observed in the *N. frontalis ENO* gene is strongly biased. Only 36 out of the 61 sense codons are used. The codons not used are always ended by A or G. Where a purine is to be found in the third position A is used in preference to G with the exception for lysine (100% AAG, 0% AAA). Filamentous fungal genes which are expressed at low level show much less codon bias than highly expressed genes (8). The codon usage observed in the *N. frontalis ENO* gene indicates a high level of expression.

Table 11.1 COMPARISON OF INTRON CHARACTERISTICS IN
MASTIGOMYCOTINAE GENES

gene	Splicing borders 5'	3'	length (bp)	G+C%
BSIKINA	GTACGC	TAG	57	64.9
	GTACTT	TAG	69	71
	GTACGT	TAG	63	60.3
BSIPROKINA	GTACGC	TAG	62	62.9
PHTTRPI	GTGCGC	CGC	171	51.5
ENO	GTAAGT	TAG	337	14.2
Consensus	GTANGT	PyAG	<100 maximum 323	

The consensus sequences are from Gurr *et al.* (8). BSIKINA: gene for the catalytic subunit of cAMP-dependent-protein kinase from *Blastocladiella emersonii* (16). BSIPROKINA: gene for the regulatory subunit of cAMP-dependent protein kinase from *Blastocladiella emersonii* (17). PHTTRPI: indole-3-glycerolphosphate synthase-N-(5' phosphoribosyl) anthranilate isomerase gene (18). ENO: *N. frontalis* enolase gene.

COMPARISON OF NUCLEOTIDE SEQUENCES

The sequences of the cDNA pPR 61 and the genomic enolase clone were compared. Sequence alignments indicated 98.7% identity between the two sequences in their coding part. Only 13 differences were observed and they did not lead to amino-acid substitution as all the differences occurred in the third position of codons. There may be two enolase genes present in *N. frontalis*. Comparisons of nucleotide sequences in the 3' non-coding part of the genomic clone and the corresponding part of the cDNA clone showed only 68.5% identity. They would support the hypothesis of two genes located in different part of the genome with different flanking sequences. On the other hand, the difference observed between one genomic clone and one cDNA clone could reveal a variant form, *i.e.* a different allele with no phenotypic effect. Very little information is available on the life cycle of *Neocallimastix* and we could not exclude an heterogenous population of nuclei in the thallus and zoospores of the fungus. Different alleles of the same gene could be present in the genomic DNA and the resulting genomic library. The presence of two *ENO* genes has been demonstrated in *S. cerevisiae* (4). The two genes and the predicted amino-acid sequences showed 95.4% identity. However, in the yeast *Candida albicans*, Brett-Mason *et al* have demonstrated the existence of a single enolase gene (5). Restriction fragment length polymorphism studies based on the differences observed in the 3' non coding part of the genomic clone and cDNA clone are needed to confirm the hypothesis of two genes in *N. frontalis.*

COMPARISONS OF ENOLASE AMINO-ACID SEQUENCES

The deduced amino-acid sequence of *N. frontalis* enolase showed a high degree of homology with sequences from enolase of other eukaryotic organisms (Fig. 11.2). Homology has been retained throughout the protein and there are numerous regions of identity among the eleven sequences analysed. The consensus sequence comprises 187 invariant amino-acids arranged in short tracts of highly conserved

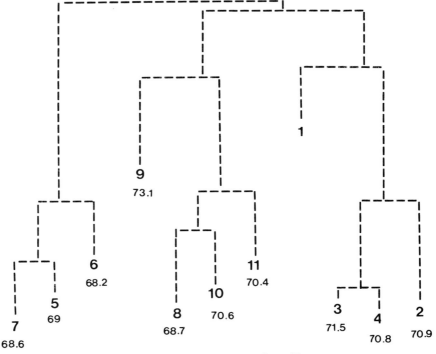

Figure 11.2. Dendrogram for the alignment of enolase amino-acid sequences
   The % of identity between *N. frontalis ENO* sequence and other sequences are shown under the branches. The best homology was found for the *Candida albicans* enolase.
   1: *N. frontalis* enolase; 2: enolase from *Candida albicans* (A45241); 3: ENO1 from *S. cerevisiae* (NOBY); 4: ENO2 from *S. cerevisiae* (NOBY2); 5: enolase from tomato (JQ1185); 6: enolase from maize (S16257); 7: enolase from *Arabidopsis* (JQ1187); 8: enolase from chicken (A23850); 9: enolase from *Drosophila* (SO7586); 10: β enolase from human (SO6756); 11: γ enolase from human (NOHUG). The numbers in brackets are the accession numbers of NBRF protein data bank.

sequences. The enolase sequences most similar to *N. frontalis* enolase are those of the yeasts *S. cerevisiae* and *C. albicans*.

The dendrogram of the alignment of enolase (Fig. 11.2) demonstrated the presence of three families. The fungal enolases (yeast, *Candida*), the plant enolases (tomato, maize, *Arabidopsis*) and animal enolases (*Drosophila*, chicken, human). In the fungal family, the enolase sequence of *N. frontalis* is clearly divergent from the yeast enolases. However, other enolase sequences from filamentous fungi are necessary to improve such comparisons in the fungal family.

Cloning and characterization of the phosphoenolpyruvate carboykinase gene (*PEPCK*)

A second cDNA originally cloned by differential screening of a cDNA library was identified by sequence homology with sequence database as a *PEPCK* gene.

NUCLEOTIDE SEQUENCE

The complete nucleotide sequence revealed an open reading frame of 1824 bp. The 3' untranslated region contains the potential AATAAA polyadenylation signal which is rarely present in fungal genes (10). The G+C content of the cDNA clone is 44.6% which is very similar to the content of the enolase gene (43.8%) and does not reflect the overall ratio for total DNA of anaerobic fungi. Codon usage observed in the *PEPCK* cDNA is largely biased; only 40 out of the 61 sense codons were used. There is a strong preference for pyrimidine and especially T in the third position of the codons. There were no differences in codon usage in the most frequently used between the *PEPCK* and the *ENO* gene codons (Table 11.2). However minor differences were that the *PEPCK* gene utilized codons for amino-acids Phe, His, Ile, Ser, Val, Tyr which were not used in the *ENO* gene. In contrast two codons for amino-acids Ala and Gly were used by *ENO* gene but not by *PEPCK* gene. The high degree of codon bias for *PEPCK* and *ENO* genes is consistent with a high level of expression of these genes, utilizing the tRNAs which are in greatest abundance in *N. frontalis*.

Table 11.2   CODON USAGE COMPARISONS IN THE *NEOCALLIMASTIX fRONTALIS* ENO GENE AND PEPCK GENE

Amino acid	Codon	No of times used NEO	No of times used PEPCK	Amino acid	Codon	No. of times used NEO	No. of times used PEPCK
Phe	UUU	0	1	Ter	UAA	1	1
	UUC	15	19		UAG	0	0
Leu	UUA	8	14	His	CAU	0	1
	UUG	0	0		CAC	6	8
	CUU	25	32				
	CUC	4	6	Gln	CAA	14	9
	CUA	0	0		CAG	0	0
	CUG	0	0				
Ile	AUU	19	19	Asn	AAU	3	5
	AUC	5	13		AAC	21	22
	AUA	0	1				
Met	AUG	9	18	Lys	AAA	0	0
					AAG	37	47
Val	GUU	26	31	Asp	GAU	22	16
	GUC	6	9		GAC	7	22
	GUA	0	0				
	GUG	0	1	Glu	GAA	29	43
					GAG	0	0
Ser	UCU	14	20	Cys	UGU	2	1
	UCC	7	11		UGC	1	5
	UCA	1	1				
	UCG	0	0	Ter	UGA	0	0
Pro	CCU	0	0	Trp	UGG	4	14
	CCC	0	0				
	CCA	17	35	Arg	CGU	11	20
	CCG	0	0		CGC	0	0
					CGA	0	0
					CGG	0	0
Thr	ACU	15	17	Ser	AGU	3	4
	ACC	3	10		AGG	0	1
	ACA	0	0				
	ACG	0	0				
Ala	GCU	32	46	Arg	AGA	2	2
	GCC	13	6		AGG	0	0
	GCA	1	0				
	GCG	0	0				
Tyr	UAU	0	1	Gly	GGU	40	52
	UAC	12	22		GGC	1	0
					GGA	1	3
					GGG	0	0

COMPARISONS OF AMINO-ACID SEQUENCES

The *N. frontalis* PEPCK protein showed respectively 50.2%, 50.4% and 48.2% amino-acid identity with the cytosolic PEPCKs of rat, chicken and fruit-fly. Homologies were mainly found in the central region of the protein. The C and N terminal sequences showed lower homology

(11). Prediction of protein secondary structure confirmed the great structural similarity of PEPCK fungal protein with other PEPCKs.

Effect of carbon sources on expression of *N. frontalis* genes

In vitro experiments have shown that the anaerobic fungus *N. frontalis* was able to grow on mono- or disaccharides and to degrade and utilize polysaccharides (cellulose, hemicelluloses) as carbon sources.

Several cDNA clones transcribed at high level when the fungus was grown in the presence of glucose were isolated from a cDNA library. These clones probably represented the most abundant transcribed sequences present in the growing fungus.

Total RNA or poly A^+ RNA were isolated after growing the fungus on different carbon sources and the abundance of transcripts was studied by standard dot blot or Northern analysis. Three clones were used to probe the transcripts:
– pPR 61 identified as the cDNA of enolase gene
– pPR 118 identified as the cDNA of PEPCK gene
– pPR 68 which is not formally identified. A partial nucleotide sequence (about 1 kb) is available and the deduced amino-acid sequence showed a significant homology to the β-succinyl-coA-synthetase gene (*beta-SCS*) from *Trichomonas vaginalis*. The β-SCS is a soluble hydrogenosomal protein (12).

EXPRESSION OF ENO GENE

Neocallimastix frontalis enolase mRNA was detected as an abundant transcript when the fungus was grown on glucose, maltose, lactose (Table 11.3). However, the amount of ENO transcripts in Avicel (crystalline cellulose) grown mycelium was several times lower. These results are reminiscent of the 20 fold glucose mediated induction of the *S. cerevisiae ENO 2* gene (13). In *Candida albicans* levels of *ENO* transcripts were 6-fold higher in glucose grown cells that in strains grown on ethanol (5). In *N. frontalis* the polysaccharide Avicel would have the same effect on enolase transcript levels as neoglucogenic sources in yeasts. It should be stressed, however that the elevated transcription of ENO gene in glucose grown mycelium may not reflect the level of the protein or enolase activity. It has been demonstrated

Table 11.3   ANALYSIS OF *N. fRONTALIS* GENE EXPRESSION ON DIFFERENT CARBON SOURCES

mRNA level	glucose	carbon source maltose	lactose	Avicel
ENO	160	135	115	15
PEPCK	155	145	125	110

The results were computed from Northern blot densitometry analysis and corrected after rehybridization of the filter with an rRNA oligonucleotide probe.

that the level of enolase protein detected by monoclonal antibodies or the enolase activity were quite similar in glucose or ethanol grown cultures (5). This suggested that cytoplasmic level of enolase was regulated post-transcriptionally by several mechanisms.

EXPRESSION OF PEPCK GENE

The mRNA level of *PEPCK* gene was quite similar in mycelia grown on glucose, maltose, lactose or Avicel (Table 11.3). A single transcript of 2.2 kb was detected (Fig. 11.3). However, the level of mRNA was higher in mycelium grown on methylglucopyranoside which is known to be an inducer of hydrolytic enzyme synthesis. PEPCK catalyze the reversible conversion of oxaloacetate to phosphoenolpyruvate; it is the key-regulatory step in the synthesis of glucose (neoglucogenesis). In limiting conditions of growth (without glucose), the gene should be expressed at high level to provide metabolizable sugar to the cells.

When comparing the abundance of transcripts of *ENO* and *PEPCK* genes in fungi grown on cellulose (Table 11.3) it clearly appeared that the two genes have different transcriptional regulation. The growing conditions which trigger the high level of synthesis of polysaccharidases have differential effects on the levels of mRNA of genes encoding glycolytic enzymes.

Poly A^+ RNA (10 µg) was fractionated on formaldehyde agarose gel and transferred to nitrocellulose membrane.
M: culture on methylglucose
G: culture on glucose
The PEPCK cDNA (A) and the β SCS cDNA (B) were used as probes.

A   B

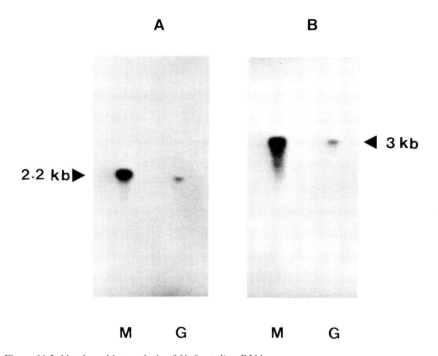

2·2 kb▶   ◀ 3 kb

M   G   M   G

Figure 11.3. Northern blot analysis of *N. frontalis* mRNA

EXPRESSION OF cDNA pPR68 CLONE

The pPR68 cDNA clone used as a probe revealed a single transcript of 3 kb which was more abundant when methylglucose was the substrate rather than glucose (Fig 11.3).

Conclusions

Two genes encoding enzymes of the glycolytic pathway have been isolated from libraries of *N. frontalis* and characterized. The G+C contents of the coding sequences of *ENO* gene and *PEPCK* gene are respectively 43.8 and 44.6%. This is in sharp contrast with the G+C content of non coding part of the genes: 14.2% for the intervening sequence of ENO gene and 15.2% and 14.2% for the 3' non coding part of *ENO* and *PEPCK* clones respectively.

Brownlee (6) stressed that the highly AT-rich genome of the anaerobic fungi might be expected to affect the amino-acid composition of the encoded proteins (6). As seen in the present studies, the amino-acid sequences of *ENO* and *PEPCK* genes showed extensive homologies with corresponding genes of various organisms (yeasts, plants, insects, mammals) and no over-abundance of those amino-acids coded for by AT rich codons was detected. The composition of the genome of *N. frontalis* would be an array of encoding sequences with normal G+C content (40, 50%) and very large intergenic non-coding regions with a high A+T content. The unique intervening sequence found in *ENO* gene is remarkably long (327 bp): this is the longest intron sequence discovered so far in filamentous fungal genes (8). The splicing rules of this intervening sequence are very similar to the splicing rules for other fungal genes. No internal consensus sequence necessary for lariat formation was found as was generally observed in other fungal genes (8). However, the presence of several repeated or inverted repeat sequences forming loops in the intervening sequence of *ENO* gene may have biological significance which has to be investigated.

The codon usages observed in the *ENO* and *PEPCK* genes of *N. frontalis* are very similar. The observed codon bias reflected the very high level of expression of these genes. Whilst regulation may undoubtedly occur at post-transcriptional levels, it is generally thought that control of filamentous fungal gene expression is exerted mainly at the stage of transcription. As seen in the present study the carbon source of the culture medium deeply affected the abundance of transcripts of *ENO* and *PEPCK* genes. Glucose and other easily metabolized sugars induced a high transcriptional level of *ENO* gene compared to the level of *ENO* transcripts detected after growth on cellulose.

The mRNA level of *PEPCK* gene was quite similar in mycelia grown on glucose or cellulose but was much enhanced when the fungus was growing on methylglucose. These studies demonstrated that the two highly expressed *ENO* and *PEPCK* genes presented different transcriptional regulations.

The study of highly expressed genes involved in basic metabolism should provide important information on promoter elements. These elements are recognized by a variety of protein factors signalling the position of transcription initiation and regulating its efficiency (14). The upstream promoting sequence of the highly expressed *ENO* gene of *N. frontalis* has been sequenced and its characterization is under study. A useful method for this purpose is the fusion of the promoter sequence (or deleted parts) to a reporter gene with an easily detectable gene product. In the few studies carried out so far with filamentous fungi, either the *lacZ* (coding for β-galactosidase) or the *uidA* (coding for β-glucuronidase) genes were used. The recombinant plasmid con-

taining *N. frontalis ENO* promoting sequences will be used for homologous transformation of *N. frontalis* and to transform different Ascomycete or Phycomycete fungal strains.

Judelson *et al* tested different promoter sequences from a range of species for activity in the Oomycetes (15). Oomycete promoters resulted in high level of glucuronidase accumulation. In contrast little or no activity was detected when promoters from higher fungi were used, indicating that the transcriptional machinery of the Oomycetes differs significantly from that of the higher fungi.

The identification and analysis of sequences regulating transcription has practical implication related to the development of vectors for gene transfer in the Phycomycetes or heterologous expression of genes from anaerobic fungi in aerobic filamentous fungi. These studies should also give new insights on the evolution of the transcriptional apparatus in fungi.

References

(1) HEBRAUD, M. and FEVRE, M. (1988). Characterization of glycoside and polysaccharide hydrolases secreted by the rumen anaerobic fungi *Neocallimastix frontalis*, *Piromonas communis* and *Sphaeromonas communis*. Journal of General Microbiology.134, 1123–1129.

(2) MARVIN-SIKKEMA, F.D., REES, E., KRAAK, M.N. GOTTSCHAL, J.C. and PRINS, R.A. (1993). Influence of metronidazole, CO, CO_2 and methanogens on the fermentative metabolism of the anaerobic fungus *Neocallimastix* sp strain L2. Applied and Environmental Microbiology. 59, 2678–2683.

(3) REYMOND, P., DURAND, R., HEBRAUD, M. and FEVRE, M. (1991). Molecular cloning of genes from the rumen anaerobic fungus *Neocallimastix frontalis:* expression during hydrolase induction. FEMS Microbiology Letters. 77, 107–112.

(4) HOLLAND, M.J., HOLLAND, J.P., THILL, G.P. and JACKSON, R.A. (1981). the primary structures of two yeast enolase genes. The Journal of Biological Chemistry. 256, 1381–1395.

(5) BRET-MASON, A., BUCKLEY, H.R. and GORMAN, J.A. (1993). Molecular cloning and characterization of the *Candida albicans* enolase gene. Journal of Bacteriology 175, 2632–2639.

(6) BROWNLEE, A.G. (1989). Remarkably A-T rich genomic

DNA from the anaerobic fungus *Neocallimastix*. Nucleic Acid Research. 17, 1327–1335.

(7)   BILLON-GRAND, G., FIOL, J.B., BRETON, A., BRUYERE, A. and OULHA, J Z. (1991). DNA of some anaerobic rumen fungi : G + C content determination. FEMS Microbiology Letters 82, 267–270.

(8)   GURR, S.J., UNKLES, S.E. and KINGHORN, J.R. (1987). The structure and organization of nuclear genes of filamentous fungi. In : Gene Structure in eukaryotic microbes (Kinghorn J.R. ed.) pp. 93–139. IRL Press Oxford.

(9)   GALLWITZ, D., HALFTER, H. and MERTINS, P. (1987). Splicing of mRNA precursors in yeast. In: Gene Structure in eukaryotic microbes (Kinghorn J.R. ed.) pp. 27–40. IRL Press Oxford

(10) UNKLES, S.E. (1992). Gene organization in industrial filamentous fungi. In: Applied molecular genetics of filamentous fungi (Kinghorn J.R. and Turner G. eds) pp. 28–53, Blakie Academic and Professional. London.

(11) REYMOND, P., GEOURJON, C., ROUX, B., DURAND, R. and FEVRE, M. (1992). Sequence of the phosphoenolpyruvate carboxykinase-encoding cDNA from the rumen anaerobic fungus *Neocallimstix frontalis*: comparison of the amino-acid sequence with animals and yeast. Gene.110, 57–63.

(12) LAHTI, C.J., OLIVEIRA, C.E. and JOHNSON, P.J. (1992). Beta-succinyl-coenzyme A synthetase from *Trichomonas vaginalis* is a soluble hydrogenosomal protein with an amino-terminal sequence that resembles mitochondrial presequences. Journal of Bacteriology. 174, 6822–6830.

(13) COHEN, R., YOKOI, T, HOLLAND, J.P., PEPPER, A.E. and HOLLAND, M.J. (1987). Transcription of the constitutively expressed yeast enolase gene ENO1 is mediated by positive and negative cis-acting regulatory sequences. Molecular and Cellular Biology. 7, 2753–2761.

(14) PUNT, P.J. and Van den HONDEL C.A.M.J.J. (1992). Analysis of transcription control sequences of fungal genes. In: Molecular signals in Plant Microbe Communication (Verma D.P.S. ed.) pp. 29–48. CRC Press Boca Raton.

(15) JUDELSON, H.S., TYLER, B.M. and MICHELMORE R.W. (1992). Regulatory sequence for expressing genes in oomycetes fungi. Molecular and General Genetics 234, 138–146.

(16) OLIVEIRA, J.F., BORGES, A.C., MARQUES, M.V. and GOMES, S.L. (1993) unpublished.

(17) LOPES-GOMES, S. and MARQUES, M. (1992). Cloning and structural analysis of the gene for the regulatory subunit of CAMP- dependent-protein kinase from *Blastocladiella emesonii*. Journal of Biological Chemistry. 267, 17201–17207.

(18) KARLOVSKY, P. and PRELL, H.N. (1991). The TRP1 of *Phytophthora parasitica* encoding indole-3-glycerolphosphate synthase -N-(5'-phosphoribosyl) anthranilate isomerase : structure and evolutionary distance from homologous fungal gene. Gene. 109, 161–165.

12

WATER-SOLUBLE POLYSACCHARIDES OF FUNGAL CELL WALLS

J.A. LEAL

Centro de Investigaciones Biológicas. CSIC. Velázquez, 144. 28006 Madrid (Spain).

Summary

Polysaccharidic fractions were obtained from fungal cell walls by alkali treatment. The polysaccharides extracted with 1M NaOH at 20°C were water-insoluble α-(1–3)-glucan or β-(1–3)-glucans (fraction F1I), and a water-soluble fraction (F1S), with different composition and structure for each genus or group of species of the same genus. The alkali resistant material is the glucan-chitin complex, which amounts to about 50% of dry cell walls.

Fraction F1S amounting from 2 to 10% of the dry cell wall material has been obtained from species of *Penicillium, Eupenicillium, Talaromyces, Paecilomyces,* and *Aspergillus.* The main component of these fractions has been purified and its composition and structure determined by gas-chromatography (gc), gas-chromatography-mass spectrometry (gc-ms) and nuclear magnetic resonance (NMR). Its distribution among the species of the genera investigated was: β-(1–5)galactofuranan in *Eupenicillium* and species of *Penicillium* and *Aspergillus;* β-(1–6)(1–5)galactofuranan in species of *Eupenicillium* and *Penicillium expansum;* a complex gluco-manno-galactan in species of *Talaromyces* and *Penicillium*; and β(1–2)(1–3)galactofuranan in species of *Talaromyces* and *Penicillium.*

The water-soluble polysaccharide from different isolates of *Paecilomyces variotii* was a β-(1–5)(1–6)galactofuranan with (1–6) and (1–2,6)mannopyranose and from *P. fumosoroseus* a β-(1–4, 6)mannopyranose and terminal galactopyranose.

The water-soluble polysaccharides may be used as chemotaxonomic characters for grouping species and for establishing relationships among species of *Penicillium* and *Paecilomyces* and their teleomorphic genera.

Introduction

Fungal cell walls are mainly composed of polysaccharides. Microfibrils of chitin or cellulose are the skeletal components which are cemented by glucans, mannans, galactans, xylans, heteropolysaccharides and proteins. The early literature on fungal cell wall chemistry has been reviewed by Aronson (1), Bartnicki-García (5), Taylor and Cameron (39) and Rosenberger (35). The structure and chemistry of fungal polysaccharides have been also reviewed (4, 17).

The fungi may be subdivided into various categories which could reach the genus level according to the chemical nature of the walls (5). The knowledge of cell wall composition is slowly advancing as a result of the application of polysaccharides in taxonomy.

New polysaccharides have been isolated from fungal cell walls. Nigeran, a hot water-soluble, cold water-insoluble α-(1–3)(1–4)-glucan of the cell wall (3) was considered a potential phylogenetic marker for *Aspergillus* and *Penicillium* species (7).

Galactofuranosyl residues have been reported in the cell walls of *P. charlesii* (10) and *P. ochrochloron* (30). The analysis of the cell wall and polysaccharidic fractions of species of *Penicillium* (24), *Eupenicillium* (13) and *Talaromyces* (37) revealed two types of cell walls: type A, has a high content of glucose and low galactose, while type B has a high content of galactose. Cell walls of type A were found in *E. crustaceum* and type B in *T. flavus*, the type species of these genera (14). Hetero-polysaccharides rich in galactofuranose were isolated and partially characterized from the cell wall of *P. erythromellis* (36) and *T. helicus* (34). Alkali and water-soluble galacto-manno-glucans were isolated from the cell walls of *Gliocladium viride* (15). Alkali and water-soluble polysaccharides have been isolated and characterized from the cell walls of fungi belonging to several genera (2, 26, 27, 31, 32).

The differences in chemical composition and structure of the water-soluble polysaccharides indicate that each genus may have its own characteristic polysaccharide. In this work it will be shown that poly-saccharides can be used as chemotaxonomic characters at the genus or subgenus level and they may help in establishing relationships among anamorphic genera and their teleomorphs.

Materials and methods

FUNGAL GROWTH

The effects of the culture media and growth conditions on fungal cell wall composition have received little attention. The content of glucose and glucosamine does not change during the incubation period once they have been incorporated into the wall polymers of *Aspergillus clavatus* (8). Glucose decreases and glucosamine increases in the cell walls of *Paecilomyces persicinum* during growth (29). The amount of the polysaccharidic fractions obtained from the cell walls of *Penicillium expansum* does not change during an incubation period of 43 days (12). The content of glucose and galactose of the cell wall of *P. allahabadense* decreases slightly during a growth period of 59 days, and the content of mannose increases (11). The amount of nigeran deposited in the cell walls of species of *Aspergillus* and *Penicillium* increases in response to nitrogen depletion (7). The mycelial and yeast forms of dimorphic fungi differ in wall composition (6, 20).

It is advisable when cell wall polysaccharides are used in chemotaxonomy that fungi should be grown under identical conditions: culture medium, agitation, temperature, time of incubation, etc. The basal medium and growth conditions for mycelium production of species of *Penicillium* and related genera were as previously described (14).

CELL WALL ISOLATION

Cell walls are obtained by mechanical disruption of the mycelium which is repeatedly washed to eliminate the cytoplasmic debris (35).

Large amounts of cell walls are obtained by disintegration of dry mycelium in a Sorvall omnimixer followed by treatment on a Fritsch 'pulverisatte 6' ball-mill. The powdered mycelium is suspended in 1% solution of sodium dodecyl sulfate containing 0.02% sodium azide and maintained in agitation overnight at 20°C. The cell wall material is collected by centrifugation at 4°C, washed with distilled water until free of cytoplasmic contamination, followed by two washes with 50% and 100% ethyl alcohol and dried at 60°C in an aerated oven. In the middle of the washing process, narrow hyphae are subjected to ultrasonic treatment to facilitate cytoplasmic release.

CELL WALL FRACTIONATION

The methods for cell wall fractionation are based on the solubility of polysaccharides in alkali or acid solutions (28). The method selected should preserve the integrity of the polysaccharides and avoid the loss of some of them. Acid treatment may destroy most polysaccharides (35). Therefore, alkali extraction should precede other treatments.

The polysaccharidic material is precipitated from the extracts with methanol, ethanol, acetone or by neutralization, and collected by centrifugation. The alkali or acid used in the extractions, and the solvents used in polysaccharide precipitation should be eliminated by dialysis since the precipitates contain water-soluble polysaccharides (36) which are lost if they are washed with water. When polysaccharides are precipitated by neutralization the water-soluble polysaccharides remain in the supernatant. They are recovered by dialysis. The extraction method used in our laboratory is shown in Fig. 12.1.

ISOLATION OF POLYSACCHARIDES FROM F1S

The water-soluble polysaccharides of fraction F1S are isolated by their different solubility in water or by gel permeation in Sepharose CL-6B using as eluent 0.3M NaOH (22).

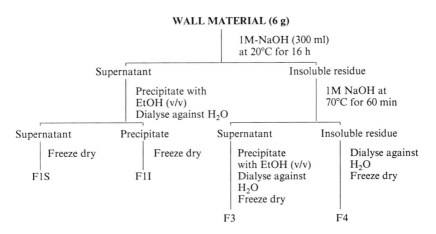

Figure 12.1. Fractionation of wall material

CHEMICAL ANALYSIS

Neutral sugars are released by hydrolysis with H_2SO_4 of different concentrations for different periods of time in sealed evacuated tubes at 100°C. The sugars are converted into their corresponding alditol acetates (21) and identified and quantified by gas-liquid chromatography (16).

METHYLATION

The procedure for the methylation analysis has been previously described (15) being basically similar to the Hakomori method (18) as modified by Jansson *et al.* (19).

NMR ANALYSIS

The polysaccharides (ca 25 mg) were dissolved in 0.7 ml of D_2O and centrifuged at 10,000 g for 15 min to remove insoluble material. ^{1}H-NMR spectra were obtained in D_2O solutions at 40°C in a Varian XL-300 spectrometer (300 MHz). The spectra were referenced to residual HDO (4.61 ppm).

Structure and distribution of water-soluble polysaccharides

β-(1–5)-GALACTOFURANAN

Fraction F1S (1.5 to 8.2% of the dry cell wall material) extracted from species of *Eupenicillium* (22, 23) is mainly composed of a β-galactofuran whose structure and conformation (25) corresponds to [-5)-Galf-β-(1-]$_n$. It has also been found in several species of *Penicillium* and *Aspergillus*, and two of *Talaromyces* (unpublished results from this laboratory). The strains of the species investigated are listed in Table 12.1 and the ^{1}H-NMR spectrum in Fig. 12.2A.

This polysaccharide may be used as a chemotaxonomic marker for the genus *Eupenicillium* since it has been found in the cell wall of most of the species analyzed. Its presence in certain species of *Penicillium* indicates that their teleomorphic state is *Eupenicillium* since the cell wall of *Talaromyces*, the other teleomorphic state of *Penicillium*, con-

Table 12.1. FUNGI CONTAINING β-(1–5)-GALACTOFURANAN IN THEIR CELL WALLS

EUPENICILLIUM	PENICILLIUM	TALAROMYCES
E. crustaceum 635.70*	*P. decumbens 258.33*	*T. emersonii 180.68*
E. angustiporcatum 202.84	*P. brevicompactum 168.44*	*T. byssochlamydoides 533.71*
E. baarnense 134.41	*P. frequentans 345.51*	
E. catenatum 352.67	*P. charmesinum 305.48*	
E. cinnamopurpureum 429.65	*P. chrysogenum 205.57*	
E. inusitatum 351.67	*P. spinulosum 269.29*	**ASPERGILLUS**
E. ochro-salmoneum 231.60	*P. erubescens 253.35*	*A. flavipes 129.61*
E. parvum 359.48	*P. oxalicum 7531-CECT*	*A. ochraceus 385.67*
E. pinetorum 235.60	*P. thomii 381.48*	*A. fumigatus RO 53*
E. shearii 290.48	*P. ingelheimense 107.66*	*A. nidulans 2544-CECT*
E. sinaicum 279.82	*P. ingelheimense 163.42*	*A. clavatus 2674-CECT*
E. stolkiae 315.67	*P. charlesii 304.48*	*A. niger 120.49*
E. terrenum 317.67	*P. allii 161.42*	*A. ornatus 385.53*
E. lapidosum 343.48	*P. atramentosum 291.48*	
	P. crustosum 313.48	
	P. hordei 701.68	

* The strains followed only by a number were from CBS.

tains β-galactofurans with different linkage types (Prieto, personal communication).

β-(1–5)(1–6)-GALACTOFURANANS

A straight chain galactan has been obtained from fraction F1S of *Eupenicillium cryptum* CBS 271.89 and three strains of *Penicillium expansum* CBS 325.48, CECT 2275 and CECT 2278 (CECT: Colección Española de Cultivos Tipo). The structure and conformation of this polysaccharide was determined (unpublished results) by gc-ms analysis of the partially methylated alditols obtained from the permethylated galactan and by ^{1}H-NMR (Fig. 2B). The repeating unit is: [-6-Galf-β-(1–5)-Galf-β-(1–5)-Galf-β-(1–5)-Galf-(1-]$_n$. It is interesting to note that the galactan of *P. expansum* differs from that of the other penicillia investigated.

A complex galactan has been isolated from several species of *Talaromyces* and *Penicillium*. The polysaccharides isolated from strains CBS 352.72 and CBS 310.38 of *T. flavus* have been investigated by chemical analysis and NMR studies (33). Two different skeletons coexist, having the structures:

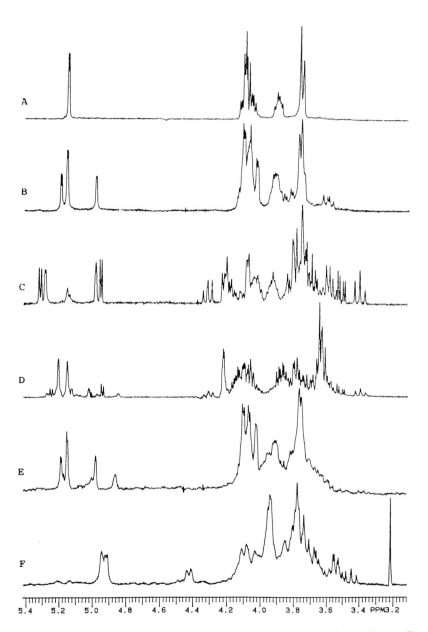

Figure 12.2. ^{1}H-NMR spectra of characteristic water-soluble polysaccharides: A) *Eupenicillium crustaceum*; B) *Penicillium expansum*; C) *Talaromyces flavus*; D) *Talaromyces wortmannii*; E) *Paecilomyces variotii*; and F) *Paecilomyces fumosoroseus*.

[-6)-β-D-Galf-(1–5)-β-D-Galf-(1-]$_n$ and   [-6-α-D-Manp-(1-]$_n$
```
              2                                        2
              ↑                                        ↑
              1                                        1
```
α-D-Glcp-(1–2)-α-D-Galf   α-D-Galf

Complex gluco-manno-galactan

The fungi in which this polysaccharide has been found are listed in Table 12.2, and the ^{1}H NMR spectrum in Fig. 12.2C. This polysaccharide may be used as chemotaxonomic marker for a large number of species of *Talaromyces*. Its presence in species of *Penicillium* shows the close relatedness between these groups of fungi.

β-(1–2)(1–3)-GALACTOFURANAN

The main component of fraction F1S of *Talaromyces wortmannii* CBS 235.38 and CBS 391.48, *T. rotundus* CBS 369.48, *Penicillium allahabadense* IJFM 1087, and *P. zacinthae* IJFM 1232 is a straight chain galactan (IJFM: Instituto Jaime Ferrán, Madrid). The linkage types were determined by gc-ms and its structure and conformation by NMR spectroscopy (Fig. 12.2D). This polysaccharide has the following repeating unit: [-3)-Galf-β-(1–2)-Galf-β-(1-]$_n$. Since the microorganisms used in this work were chosen at random it seems that this polysaccharide will be found in only a limited number of species of *Penicillium* and *Talaromyces*.

Table 12.2   FUNGI CONTAINING COMPLEX GLUCO-MANNO-GALACTAN

PENICILLIUM	TALAROMYCES
P. allahabadense 762.68	*T. flavus 352.72*
P. islandicum 338.48	*T. flavus 310.38*
P. verruculosum WA 30	*T. flavus W 36*
P. pinophilum 439.89	*T. bacillisporus 136.45*
P. purpurogenum 365.48	*T. stipitatus 375.48*
P. diversum 320.48	*T. helicus 335.48*
P. erythromellis 7284-IJFM	*T. macrosporus 117.72*
P. aculeatum 289.48	*T. mimosinus 659.80*
P. dendriticum 660.80	*T. purpureus 475.71*
P. funiculosum 2702-CECT	

GLUCOGALACTOMANNANS

These polysaccharides have been isolated from fraction F1S of two species of the genus *Paecilomyces*. The polysaccharide found in *P. variotii* CBS 323.34, CBS 990.73A, CBS 339.51 and CBS 371.60 is composed of glucose, galactose and mannose. The methyl hexitol analyzed by gc-ms revealed predominantly β-(1–5)galactofuranose β-(1–6) mannopyranose and β-(1–2, 6)mannopyranose (9). The ^{1}H-NMR spectrum is shown in Fig. 12.2E.

The polysaccharide obtained from *P. fumosoroseus* CBS 244.31, CBS 339.54, CBS 337.52 and CBS 375.70 has a composition very close to that of *P. variotii* but with different linkage types: β-(1–4,6)mannopyranose and terminal galactopyranose. The investigation of the structure and conformation of these polysaccharides is in progress. The ^{1}H-NMR spectrum is shown in Fig. 12.2F.

The results obtained in the analysis of the cell wall of these two species of *Paecilomyces* agree with traditional taxonomy since *P. variotii* belongs to section *Paecilomyces* and *P. fumosoroseus* to section *Isaroidea* (38).

It is interesting to note that the composition and structure of the polysaccharides of these species of *Paecilomyces* differ from the related genera *Eupenicillium* and *Talaromyces*. The teleomorphic state of certain species of *Paecilomyces* is *Talaromyces*.

Conclusions

The number of genera and species investigated are small and only a few water-soluble polysaccharides have been characterized to date. Nevertheless the results are encouraging and permit the following conclusions:

a) Fungal cell walls contain water-soluble polysaccharides which may have similar composition and structure for most species of a genus as in *Eupenicillium*, revealing that it is homogeneous. Other genera (*Penicillium, Talaromyces* and *Paecilomyces*) have several polysaccharides which are separately found in groups of species. This shows that these genera are heterogeneous.

b) Water-soluble polysaccharides may help to establish the relatedness of the species of anamorphic genera (*Penicillium, Paecilomyces*, etc..) with the perfect states (*Eupenicillium, Talaromyces*, etc ...). This could improve the systematics of anamorphic genera whose species could be grouped by the similarity of their wall polysaccharides with those found in their teleomorphs.

c) The water-soluble polysaccharides of the cell wall and other cell wall polysaccharides in combination with morphology, analysis of secondary metabolites, genetic studies, isoenzyme electrophoresis, etc., may be useful in the creation of natural taxa at the genus or subgenus level.

Acknowledgments

This research was supported by Grants PB 87/0243 and PB 91/0054 from Dirección General de Investigación Científica y Técnica. I am grateful to Dr. M. Bernabé for the NMR-analysis of polysaccharides and stimulating discussions and to Drs. B. Gómez-Miranda, A. Prieto, and Miss Domenech who contributed to this project.

References

(1)   ARONSON, J.M. (1965). In: The Fungi. Vol. I. The fungal cell. (Ainsworth G.C. and Sussman, A.S. eds) Academic Press. New York and London, pp. 49–76.

(2)   BARDALAYE, P.C. and NORDIN, J.H. (1977). Chemical structure of the galactomannan from the cell wall of *Aspergillus niger*. Journal of Biological Chemistry 252, 2584–2591.

(3)   BARKER, S.A., BOURNE, E.J., OMANT, D.M. and STACEY, M. (1957). Studies of *A. niger*. Part. VI. The separation and structures of oligosaccharides from nigeran. Journal of the Chemical Society. 2448–2454.

(4)   BARRETO-BERGTER, E., and GORIN, P.A.J. (1983). Structural chemistry of polysaccharides from fungi and lichens. Advances in Carbohydrate Chemistry and Biochemistry 41, 67–103.

(5)   BARTNICKI-GARCIA, S. (1968). Cell wall chemistry, morphogenesis, and taxonomy of fungi. Annual Review of Microbiology 22, 87–108.

(6)   BARTNICKI-GARCIA, S. and NICKERSON, W.S. (1962). Isolation, composition and structure of cell walls of filamentous and yeast-like forms of *Mucor rouxii*. Biochimica et Biophysica Acta 58, 102–119.

(7)   BOBBITT, F., and NORDIN, J.H. (1978). Hyphal nigeran as a potential phylogenetic marker for *Aspergillus* and *Penicillium* species. Mycologia 70, 1201–1211.

(8) CORINA, D.L. and MUNDAY, K.A. (1971). The metabolic stability of carbohydrates in walls of hyphae of *Aspergillus clavatus*. Journal of General Microbiology 65, 253–257.

(9) DOMENECH, J., PRIETO, A., BERNABE, M. and LEAL, J.A. (1994). Cell wall polysaccharides of four strains of *Paecilomyces variotii*. Current Microbiology 28, 169–173.

(10) GANDER, J.E., JENTOFT, N.H.,, DREWES, L.R. and RICK, P.D. (1974). The 5-O-β-D-galactofuranosyl-containing exocellular glycopeptide of *Penicillium charlesii*. Characterization of the phosphogalactomannan. Journal of Biological Chemistry 249, 2063–1072.

(11) GOMEZ-MIRANDA, B., GUERRERO, C. and LEAL, J.A. (1984). Effect of culture age on cell wall polysaccharides of *Penicillium allahabadense*. Experimental Mycology 8, 298–303.

(12) GOMEZ-MIRANDA, B., and LEAL, J.A. (1985). Carbohydrate stability during ageing in *Penicillium expansum* cell wall. Microbiología SEM 1, 67–75.

(13) GOMEZ-MIRANDA, B., MOYA, A. and LEAL, J.A. (1986). Hyphal polysaccharides as potential phylogenetic markers for *Eupenicillium* species. Experimental Mycology 10, 184–189.

(14) GOMEZ-MIRANDA, B., MOYA, A., and LEAL, J.A. (1988). Differences in the cell wall composition in the type species of *Eupenicillium* and *Talaromyces*. Experimental Mycology 12, 258–263.

(15) GOMEZ-MIRANDA, B., PRIETO, A. and LEAL, J.A. (1990). Chemical composition and characterization of a galactomannoglucan from *Gliocladium viride* wall material. FEMS Microbiology Letters 70, 331–336.

(16) GOMEZ-MIRANDA, B., RUPEREZ, P. and LEAL, J.A. (1981). Changes in chemical composition during germination of *Botrytis cinerea*. Current Microbiology 6, 243–246.

(17) GORIN, P.A.J. and SPENCER, J.E.T., (1968). Structural chemistry of fungal polysaccharides. Advances in Carbohydrate Chemistry 23, 367–417.

(18) HAKOMORI, S.I. (1964). A rapid permethylation of glycolipid and polysaccharide catalysed by methylsulfinyl carbanion in dimethyl sulfoxide. Journal of Biochemistry (Tokio) 55, 205–208.

(19) JANSSON, P.-E., KENNE, L., LIEDGREN, H., LINDBERG, B. and LÖNNGREN, J. (1976). A practical guide to the methylation analysis of carbohydrates. Chem. Commun. Univ. Stockholm. 8.

(20) KANETSUNA, F., and CARBONELL, L.M. (1970). Cell wall glucans of the yeast and mycelial forms of *Paracoccidoides brasiliensis*. Journal of Bacteriology 101, 675–680.

(21) LAINE, R.A., ESSELMAN, W.J. and SWEELEY, C.C. (1972). Gas-liquid chromatography of carbohydrates. In: Methods in Enzymology 28 (Colowick, S.P. and Kaplan, N.O., eds) pp. 159–167. Academic Press, N.Y.-London.

(22) LEAL, J.A., GOMEZ-MIRANDA, B., PRIETO, A. and BERNABE, M. (1993). Differences in cell wall polysaccharides of several species of *Eupenicillium*. FEMS Microbiology Letters 108, 341–346.

(23) LEAL, J.A., GUERRERO, C., GOMEZ-MIRANDA, B., PRIETO, A. and BERNABE, M. (1992). Chemical and structural similarities in wall polysaccharides of some *Penicillium, Eupenicillium* and *Aspergillus* species. FEMS Microbiology Letters 90, 165–168.

(24) LEAL, J.A., MOYA, A., GOMEZ-MIRANDA, B., RUPEREZ, P. and GUERRERO, C. (1984). Differences in cell wall polysaccharides in some species of *Penicillium*. In: Cell Wall Synthesis and Autolysis (Nombela, C. ed.). pp. 149–155. Elsevier Science Publishers: Amsterdam/New York.

(25) LEAL, J.A., PRIETO, A., GOMEZ-MIRANDA, B., JIMENEZ-BARBERO, J. and BERNABE, M. (1993). Structure and conformational features of an alkali- and water-soluble galactofuranan from the cell walls of *Eupenicillium crustaceum*. Carbohydrate Research 244, 361–368.

(26) LLOYD, K.O. (1970). Isolation, characterization and partial structure of peptido galactomannans from the yeast form of *Cladosporium werneckii*. Biochemistry 9, 3446–3453.

(27) LLOYD, K.O. (1972). Molecular organization of a covalent peptido-phosphopolysaccharide complex from the yeast form of *Cladosporium werneckii*. Biochemistry 11, 3884–3890.

(28) MAHADEVAN, P.R. and TATUM, E.L. (1965). Relationship of the major constituents of the *Neurospora crassa* cell wall to wild-type and colonial morphology. Journal of Bacteriology 90, 1073–1081.

(29) MALOWITZ, R. and PISANO, M.A. (1982). Changes in cell wall carbohydrate composition of *Paecilomyces persicinus* P-10 M1 during growth and cephalosporin C production. Applied and Environmental Microbiology 43, 916–923.

(30) MATSUNAGA, T., OKUBO, A., FUKAMI, M., YAMAZI, S.

and TODA, S. (1981). Identification of β-galactofuranosyl residues and their rapid internal motion in the *Penicillium ochrochloron* cell wall probed by ^{13}C-NMR. Biochemical and Biophysical Research Communications 102, 502–530.

(31)   NAKAJIMA, T., SASAKI, H., SATO, M., TAMARI, K., and MATSUDA, K. (1977). A cell wall proteo-heteroglycan from *Piricularia oryzae*: further studies of the structure. Journal of Biochemistry 82, 1657–1662.

(32)   NAKAJIMA, T., YOSHIDA, M., NAKAMURA, M., HIURA, N., and MATSUDA, K. (1984). Structure of the cell wall proteogalactomannan from *Neurospora crassa*. II. Structural analysis of the polysaccharide part. Journal of Biochemistry 96, 1013–1020.

(33)   PARRA, E., JIMENEZ-BARBERO, J., BERNABE, M., LEAL, J.A., PRIETO, A. and GOMEZ-MIRANDA, B. (1994). Structural studies of fungal cell-wall polysaccharides from two strains of *Talaromyces flavus*. Carbohydrate Research 251, 351–325.

(34)   PRIETO, A., RUPEREZ, P., HERNANDEZ-BARRANCO, A., and LEAL, J.A. (1988). Partial characterisation of galactose-containing heteropolysaccharides from the cell walls of *Talaromyces helicus*. Carbohydrate Research 177, 265–272.

(35)   ROSENBERGER, R.E. (1976). The cell wall. In: The Filamentous Fungi. Vol. II Biosynthesis and metabolism. (Smith, J.E. and Berry, D.R. eds.) Edward Arnold (Publishers) pp. 328–344.

(36)   RUPEREZ, P. and LEAL, J.A. (1987). Mannoglucogalactans from the cell walls of *Penicillium erythromellis*: isolation and partial characterization. Carbohydrate Research 167, 269–278.

(37)   RUPEREZ, P., MOYA, A. and LEAL, J.A. (1986). Cell wall polysaccharides from *Talaromyces* species. Archives of Microbiology 146, 250–255.

(38)   SAMSON, R.A. (1974). *Paecilomyces* and some allied hyphomycetes. Studies in Mycology, Baarn 6, 1–119.

(39)   TAYLOR, I.F.P. and CAMERON, D.S. (1973). Preparation and quantitative analysis of fungal cell walls. Strategy and tactics. Annual Review of Microbiology 27, 243–260.

13

CELL WALL COMPOSITION AND DETECTION OF ANAEROBIC RUMEN FUNGI *IN VIVO* USING FLUORESCENT LECTINS

A. BRETON[1], M. DUSSER[2], B. GAILLARD-MARTINIE[1] and J. GUILLOT[2]

[1]*Laboratoire de Microbiologie, INRA, Centre de Recherches de Clermont-Ferrand-Theix, 63122 Saint-Genès-Champanelle, France*
[2] *Laboratoire de Botanique et Cryptogamie, Faculté de Pharmacie, Université Clermont I, 63000 Clermont-Ferrand, France*

Summary

The technique based on fluorescein linked lectins was used to determine the cell wall surface composition of anaerobic rumen fungi to genera *Neocallimastix*, *Piromyces*, *Caecomyces*, *Orpinomyces* and *Anaeromyces*, appears to be an interesting tool for distinguishing between strains. Furthermore, this technique shows differences in cell wall composition between different parts of the thallus (sporangia, rhizoïds, vesicles). Positive reaction could be observed with some D-arabinose/L-fucose, *N*-acetyl-D-galactosamine, diacetylchitobiose, or oligosaccharides with a terminal galactose bound to *N*-acetylgalactosamine or *N*-acetylglucosamine by β1→3 bond-specific lectins.

Fluorescent lectins have revealed to be a valuable means of detecting rumen fungi adhering *in vivo* to plant particles and of following what becomes of them during intestinal passage and in faeces.

Introduction

Lectins are either proteins or glycoproteins of non-immune origin, able to link with sugars, agglutinate cells and/or precipitate glycoconjugates (3). They were first found in plants and then in fungi, but also exist in vertebrates, invertebrates and even on the surface of bacteria. Class I lectins (exolectins) recognize monosaccharides and are therefore inhibited by simple sugars. Class II lectins (endolectins) do not recognize a specific monosaccharide but an oligosaccharide sequence.

Due to the property of lectins which enables them to link specifically with carbohydrate molecules, glycoproteins or glycolipids, they can be put to use in various ways. This specificity can allow the isolation of glycoconjugates in the membrane or in solution, the separation of cells such as lymphocytes, microbiological diagnosis such as the characterization of trypanosoma (4) or yeasts (5), the determination of the number of receptors on the cell surface and also the visualization of cell carbohydrate molecules by labelling with fluorescent lectins combined either with fluorescein isothiocyanate (FITC) or with rhodamine tetramethyl isothiocyanate, or by the application of immuno-fluorescence techniques.

Lectins have also been used as a tool for studying the cell wall sugar composition of anaerobic fungi in the digestive tract of herbivores and also for attempting to find new criteria for the identification of strains which are both very morphologically similar and of great variability according to the age of the cultures and environmental conditions. Furthermore, fluorescence microscopy has revealed itself to be a valuable means of detecting rumen fungi adhering *in vivo* to food particles and of following what becomes of them during intestinal passage.

Cell wall composition of anaerobic rumen fungi

MATERIALS AND METHODS

Lectins, combined with fluorescein isothiocyanate and chosen according to their specificity, were used for labelling cell wall components due to their ability to recognize carbohydrate sequences. They come from basidiomycete fungi and higher plant seeds (7). Their origin, specificity and inhibitory sugars are reported in Table 13.1. They were used to identify the sugars present on the surface of whole thalli or on semi-thin sections.

Thalli cultivated on Orpin's medium (9) or on Lowe's medium (8) were separated by centrifugation, washed with 0.01 M PBS buffer (pH = 7.2) and then placed between slide and coverslip. A drop of lectin solution was placed on one of the borders of the coverslip under which it diffused, creating a concentration gradient. Observations were made with a fluorescence microscope after 20 minutes of contact in darkness at 4°C in a moist room. The binding specificity was confirmed using a lectin solution mixed with an equal volume of a 0.1M solution of inhibitory (hapteric) sugar.

Table 13.1 LECTINS USED AND THEIR CORRESPONDING INHIBITORY SUGARS

Lectin	Sources	Carbohydrate specificities	Inhibitory sugars
DSL	*Datura stramonium*	(D-Glc-*N*Ac)2	D-Glc*N*Ac
WGA	*Triticum vulgare*	(D-Glc-*N*Ac)2, sialic acid	D-Glc*N*Ac
SBA	*Glycine max*	a-D-Gal*N*Ac, β-D-Gal*N*Ac	D-Gal*N*Ac
SJL	*Sophora japonica*	D-Gal β1 → 3 D-Gal*N*Ac	D-Gal*N*Ac
LDL	*Lactarius deliciosus*	D-Gal β1 → 3 D-Gal*N*Ac	D-Gal*N*Ac
LAF	*Laccaria amethystina*	L-Fuc, D-Arab	L-Fuc
PSL	*Pholiota squarrosa*	L-Fuc, D-Arab	L-Fuc
CGL	*Clitocybe geotropa*	L-Fuc, D-Arab	L-Fuc

The semi-thin sections (0.5 µm), set in Epon resin, were treated with Maxwell solution for 3 to 4 minutes, rinsed with PBS/methanol and with PBS, then put into contact with the labelled lectin for 1/2 hour at 4°C, washed with PBS and observed with a fluorescence microscope. Indirect immunofluorescence techniques had also been considered for use in studying cell wall sugar composition (1) by treating semi-thin sections with non-labelled lectins, anti-lectin rabbit immunoserums and goat anti-bodies against rabbit anti IgG labelled with FITC. Because of the non-specific adhesion of the rabbit anti-bodies on the fungi, it was impossible to exploit the results or to transpose this method for use in an electron microscopy examination.

STRAIN CELL WALL COMPOSITION OF DIFFERENT SPECIES

The labelling of the cell walls of fungi in a pure culture (Plates I, II) was achieved through use of fluorescent lectins specific for chitobiose, D-arabinose/L-fucose, *N*-acetyl-D-galactosamine and oligosaccharides with a galactose terminal linked with a β1→3 bond either with *N*-acetylglucosamine or with *N*-acetylgalactosamine. The results obtained are reported in Table 13.2.

The presence of chitobiose, established in rumen fungi by Orpin (10), was revealed by a reactivity to wheat lectin (**WGA**) and that of *Datura* (**DSL**). The comparison of the results obtained (Table 13.2) with these two lectins showed differences, as in the case of *Piromyces mae* rhizoids and *Piromyces dumbonica* thalli, that can be explained by accessibility characters perhaps in reference to the molecular weight of the lectins.

Furthermore the same observation is also valid for *Laccaria amethystina* (**LAF**) and *Pholiota squarrosa* (**PSL**) lectins specific for

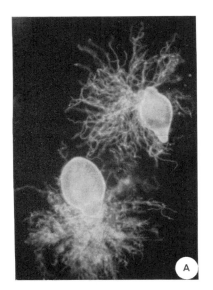

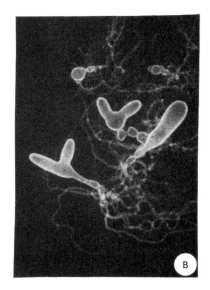

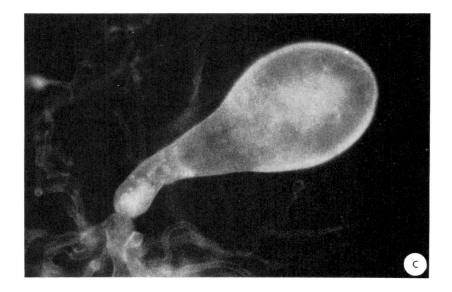

Plate I: Rumen fungi in pure culture, labelled with lectins
A: *Piromyces dumbonica* (WGA) × 400
B: *Piromyces mae* (WGA) × 400
C: *Piromyces mae* (SBA) × 1500

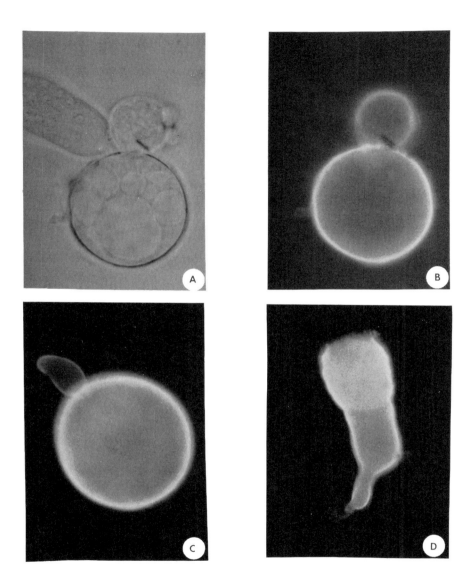

Plate II: Rumen fungi in pure culture, labelled with lectins
A: *Caecomyces communis*: sporangium and vesicles without lectin × 1400
B: *Caecomyces communis*: the same thallus (SBA) Note, no fluorescence of the sporangium
   × 1400
C: *Caecomyces communis*: young thallus (DSL) × 1400
D: *Neocallimastix sp*: sporangiophore and sporangium after zoospores release (PSL) × 1500

Table 13.2   CELL WALL COMPOSITION OF STRAINS FROM DIFFERENT SPECIES

Specific carbohydrates *Lectins*	*Chitobiose (D-glc-Nac)₂*		*D-arabinose L-fucose*		*N-acetyl galactosamine*	*D-Galβ1→3D-GalNAc*
	WGA	*DSL*	*LAF*	*PSL*	*SBA*	*SJL-LDL*
Piromyces						
P. communis (FL)						
sporangia		−	+		+	+
sporangiophores	nd	nd	+	nd	+	−
rhizoids		−	−		−	. −
P. communis (A8)						
sporangia		±	−		+	+
sporangiophores	nd	±	−	nd	−	+
rhizoids		−	−		−	−
P. mae (T1A9)						
sporangia	+	−	±	−	+	−
rhizoids	+	−	+	−	+	−
P. mae (9)						
sporangia	+	−	+	−	+	−
rhizoids	+	−	+	−	+	−
P. rhizinflata						
sporangia	nd	+	+	−	+	−
rhizoids		−	+	−	+	−
P. dumbonica						
sporangia	+	−	−	−	+	−
rhizoids	+	−	±	−	+	−
Caecomyces						
C. communis						
sporangia	nd	+	−	−	+	−
vesicles		+	+	−	+	−
C. equi						
sporangia	nd	+	−	−	+	−
vesicles		+	+	−	+	−
Neocallimastix						
N. frontalis MCH3						
sporangia	nd	−	+	+	±	nd
rhizoids		−	+	±	±	
N. variabilis						
sporangia	+	nd	nd	+	nd	nd
rhizoids	+		−			
Anaeromyces						
A. mucronatus						
sporangia	nd	−	−	−	−	nd
rhizomycelium		−	+	−	+	
Orpinomyces						
Orpinomyces joyonii						
sporangia	nd	−	+	+	−	nd
rhizomycelium		±	±	−	−	

nd: no determined, (-): no fluorescence, (±): low intensity of fluorescence, (+): high intensity of fluorescence

D-arabinose and L-fucose which can give opposite reactions; LAF, of a small size (MW = 16000), would be an optional exolectin (6). An analysis of the cell walls of a strain of *Caecomyces communis* carried out by GC on silicoa gel (results un-published) revealed the absence of L-fucose and the presence of D-arabinose. This sugar, detected by LAF lectin, is present on the surface of most of the strains studied. *Neocalli-mastix* and *Orpinomyces*, the only to react species to PSL lectin, would possess arabinose at the bottom of the chain.

N-acetylgalactosamine recognized by soya lectin (SBA) is a component of the cell walls of almost all of the strains studied.

D-galactose linked with *N*-acetylglucosamine or *N*-acetylgalactosa-mine, recognized by *Sophora* lectins (SJL) and lectins of different species of *Lactarius* amongst which is *Lactarius deliciosus* (LDL), is, on the other hand, a wall surface component characteristic of *Piromyces communis*, and lacking in all other *Piromyces* and *Caecomyces*.

Studies conducted under fluorescence microscopy on semi-thin sections of *Caecomyces communis* (1) treated with DSL,SBA and LAF showed that these three lectins can adhere to both sporangia and vesicles, thus revealing, differences in their cell wall structure. The sporangium cell wall does, in fact, include an external layer to which the three tested lectins adhered and an internal layer which remained unlabelled and is therefore of a different composition; the vesicle wall, however, presents only the lectin reactive layer and would therefore seem to be continuous with the external wall zone of the sporangia.

COMPARATIVE CELL WALL COMPOSITION OF SPORANGIA, RHIZOÏDS AND VESICLES

Upon examination of Table 13.2 it is revealed that differences in reactivity to lectins can exist between sporangia, rhizoïds or vesicles of the same strain, as is the case for *Piromyces communis* whose sporangia and rhizoïds have opposite reactions to soya lectin (SBA), *P. rhizinflata* as regards *Datura* lectin (DSL), and also for *Caecomyces communis* with SBA lectin of which only vesicles are fluorescent (Plate II, A, B). However, the inverse behaviour between morphological structures of a same thallus does not always seem to be the result of marked differences in the sugar composition of their cell walls; it could be the expression of differences in molecular sequences containing certain accessible or inaccessible sugars, according to the case, and their specific lectins. Thus, with certain *Piromyces*, chitobiose, which always binds wheat lectin (WGA), occasionally does not bind *Datura* lectin (DSL).

Reactivity to lectins appears to be far more constant for rhizoïds than for sporangia for which the intensity of the fluorescence can be a function of the state of differentiation. Thus, *P. mae* sporangia, with soya lectin, are much more fluorescent in their young state than at maturity.

TAXONOMIC CONSEQUENCES OF REACTIVITY TO LECTINS

The genera of anaerobic fungi can presently be well defined on the bases of the monocentric or polycentric characteristics of the thallus, the nature of the vegetative apparatus (rhizoïdal or vesicular) and the uni or pluriflagellate nature of the zoospores, the species are, however, sometimes difficult to identify because of their variability and of the small number of morphological characteristics, such as those of the genera *Neocallimastix* and *Piromyces*. Can lectins form a criteria of identification for anaerobic fungi?

On a generic level, it is remarkable that only *Neocallimastix* and *Orpinomyces* react positively to *Pholiota squarrosa* lectin (Plate II, D), contrary to the numerous strains of *Piromyces*, *Caecomyces* and *Anaeromyces* that were tested.

On a specific level, the compared analyses of the profiles obtained for the genus *Piromyces*, the most studied, ellicits various observations. As regards *Piromyces communis* (sporangia frequently highly pedicellated, exogenous sporangial development), the positive reactivity to *Sophora* and *Lactarius* lectins reveals the presence, on the sporangial wall surface, of D-Gal $\beta 1 \rightarrow 3$ D-Glc *N*Ac or D-Gal*N*Ac, contrary to other *Piromyces*.

Furthermore, the great differences existing between the profiles of the two strains of *Piromyces communis* that were studied lead us to believe that they could be of two different species. Last of all, the inverse reactivities that occur for SBA, SJL and LDL lectins between the *Piromyces communis* sporangia and sporangiophores mean that these structures, above and beyond their different functions, are two distinct entities on a cytological level. As for *P. mae*, *P. rhizinflata* and *P. dumbonica* (sporangia with no or only short sporangiophore, endogenous sporangial development), their identical reactivity to all tested lectins, except to those of *Datura* and soya, confirm their close taxonomic similarity.

The study of various strains of *Caecomyces* showed great homogeneity in their reaction to lectins, contrary to *Neocallimastix* which forms a complex genus whose strains, and probably even species, are highly diverse.

Application in the detection of anaerobic fungi *in vivo*

During their life cycle fungi adhere to plant fragments, in the cow or sheep rumen for example, in order to degrade their cell wall components. In order to observe this colonization, or to follow the evolution of fungal microorganisms during intestinal passage and in the faeces, fluorescent lectins were used to label their cell walls (2). The samples, which can be taken at different points along the digestive track in fistulated animals or after slaughter, were placed on a filter and rinsed with PBS buffer, then transferred to haemolysis tubes with a drop of wheat germ lectin (WGA) labelled with FITC. After 20 minutes contact at 4°C, the samples were washed and observed under fluorescence microscopy (plate III, B, C, D). *Pholiota squarrosa* lectin (PSL) labelling was also carried out to detect *Neocallimastix* for which this lectin revealed itself to be specific (plate III, B). The fungi can also be obtained by introducing, into the rumen or duodenum of fistulated animals, nylon bags (20–50 mesh) containing, for example, maize stalk, lucerne stem or soya bean pellicle fragments. After 24 or 48 hours of *in vivo* incubation, the plant fragments were rinsed with PBS buffer and then treated as before with lectin which allows, under fluorescence, a better visualization of tissue colonization by the adhering fungi (plate III, A).

Conclusion

The usage of lectins has made it possible to reveal the presence, on the surface of anaerobic fungi, of chitobiose, fucose-arabinose and *N*-acetylgalactosamine. When used on sections of *Caecomyces communis* they revealed the existence of two layers at sporangial cell wall level, of which only the outer one, continuous with the vesicle cell wall, allows them to adhere. The choice of different lectins specific for a same sugar and therefore prone to inverse reaction according to its position, has proven to be useful in differentiating certain strains. The differences in reactivity towards lectins between rhizoids or vesicles, sporangia and

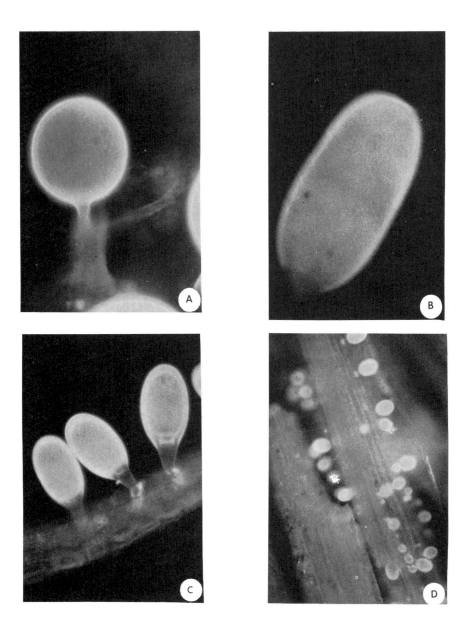

Plate III: Rumen fungi on plant particles, labelled with lectins
A: *Neocallimastix joyonii* from cow rumen (CGL) × 1400
B: *Neocallimastix sp* from sheep rumen (PSL) × 1500
C: Sporangia from sheep duodenum (WGA) × 750
D: Colonization on plant particles with sporangia from sheep duodenum (WGA) × 350

sporangiophores also contributes to the diversification of profiles. The usage of lectins which recognize oligosaccharide sequences instead of simple sugars only, as is the case for *Sophora* and *Lactarius* lectins which specifically bound to *Piromyces communis,* should facilitate the identification of certain taxons. The genus *Neocallimastix* appears as having highly diverse strains, and probably species, but they all have in common their positive reaction to *Pholiota squarrosa* lectin. The genus *Piromyces* could be consisted of two group species according to their reactivity or non-reactivity to *Sophora* and *Lactarius* lectins. Within the genus *Caecomyces* there is great homogeneity in reactivity. These results require development through the study of a greater number of strains in order to appreciate the degree of homogeneity within the species.

References

(1)   BAYARD, C. (1990). Etude de la paroi de *Caecomyces communis,* champignon anaérobie du rumen á l'aide de lectines. Mémoire de Diplôme d'Etudes Approfondies. Université de Clermont-Ferrand II.

(2)   CONFESSON, I. (1992). Etude descriptive et expérimentale de la survie des champignons anaérobies dans le tube digestif de mouton et dans le milieu extérieur. Mémoire de Diplôme d'Etudes Approfondies. Université de Clermont-Ferrand II.

(3)   GOLDSTEIN, I.J., HUGHES, R.C., MONSIGNY, M., OSAWA, T. and SHARON, N. (1980). What should be called a lectin? Nature, 66, vol. 285.

(4)   GUEUGNOT, J. (1980). Recherches sur la valeur des lectines dans l'étude taxonomique de *Trypanosomatidae des genres Chrithidia, Blastocrithidia, Leishmania, Trypanosoma.* Thèse de Doctorat d'Etat. 224 Pages. Université de Clermont-Ferrand I.

(5)   GUILLOT, J., SCANDARIATO, M. and COULET, M. (1974). Agglutinating properties of lectins as taxonomic test for *Candida* species. Annales de Microbiologie, 125B, 489–500.

(6)   GUILLOT, J., GENAUD, L., GUEUGNOT, J. and DAMEZ, M. (1983). Purification and properties of two hemagglutins of the mushroom *Laccaria amethystina.*

(7)   GUILLOT, J., BRETON, A., DAMEZ, M., DUSSER, M., GAILLARD, B. and MILLET, L. (1990). Use of lectins for a

comparative study of cell wall composition of different anaerobic rumen fungal strains. FEMS Microbiol. Lett., 65, 151–156.

(8)   LOWE, S.E., THEODOROU, M.K., TRINCI, A.P.J. and HESPELL, R.B. (1985). Growth of anaerobic rumen fungi on defined and semi-defined media lacking rumen fluid. J. Gen. Microbiol., 131, 2225–2229.

(9)   ORPIN, C.G. (1975). Studies on the rumen flagellate *Neocallimastix frontalis.* J. Gen. Microbiol., 91, 249–262.

(10) ORPIN, C.G. (1977). The occurence of chitin in the cell walls of the rumen organisms *Neocallimastix frontalis, Piromonas communis* and *Sphaeromonas communis.* J. Gen. Microbiol., 99, 215–218.

14

HYDROGENOSOMES OF THE ANAEROBIC FUNGUS
NEOCALLIMASTIX sp. L2.

R.A. PRINS, F.D. MARVIN-SIKKEMA, M. VAN DER GIEZEN
and J.C. GOTTSCHAL
*Department of Microbiology, University of Groningen, P.O. Box 14,
9750 AA Haren, The Netherlands*

Summary

The pathway of glucose catabolism in the strictly anaerobic fungus
Neocallimastix sp. L2 was studied by assaying its enzymes in whole
cell-free extracts, cytosolic and hydrogenosomal fractions. Taken
together with evidence from labelling studies the results strongly suggest that the initial glucose catabolism proceeds via the Emden-Meyer-
hof-Parnas pathway. Furthermore, all enzymes catalyzing the
conversions of phosphoenolpyruvate to acetylCoA plus formate, lactate, ethanol and succinate were found in the cytosol.

Hydrogenosomes contain enzymes involved in the oxidation of
malate to acetylCoA, carbon dioxide and hydrogen. The hydrogenosome fraction also contained an adenylate kinase activity and an
ATPase, while strong evidence was obtained for the presence of an
ADP/ATP translocase at the hydrogenosomal membrane. The ATPase
is not inhibited by the classical mitochondrial ATPase-inhibitors, but
only by diethylstilbestrol (DES). Measurements with the fluorescent
probe BCECF indicated that the interior of the hydrogenosome is
alkaline *versus* the outside of the organelle. The $\triangle$pH could be abolished after pretreatment with DES, suggesting that the ATPase is
involved in the generation of the $\triangle$pH.

On the basis of these studies a scheme was proposed for the complete
route of glucose catabolism (Fig. 14.1). In this scheme phosphoenolpyruvate is either channelled via pyruvate to acetylCoA in the cytosol,
or is channelled via malate to the hydrogenosome.

Malate is the chief substrate for the hydrogenosomes and pyruvate is
an intermediate in malate oxidation. Energy in acetylCoA can be used

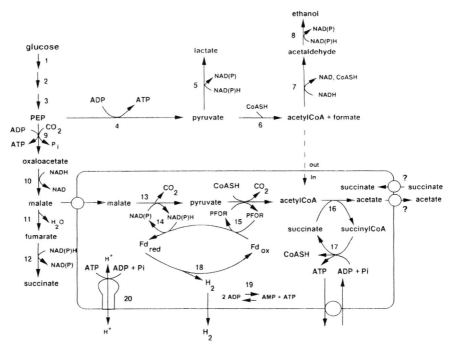

Figure 14.1. Pathway of glucose catabolism in *Neocallimastix* sp. L2. Reactions within the box are carried out within hydrogenosomes.

Enzymes detected: 1 = hexokinase; 2 = phosphofructokinase; 3 = enolase; 4 = pyruvate kinase; 5 = lactate dehydrogenase; 6 = pyruvate formate lyase; 7 = acetaldehyde dehydrogenase; 8 = alcohol dehydrogenase; 9 = PEP carboxylase and PEP carboxykinase; 10 = malate dehydrogenase; 11 = fumarase; 12 = fumarate reductase; 13 = malic enzyme; 14 = NAD(P)H:ferredoxin oxidoreductase; 15 = pyruvate:ferredoxin oxidoreductase; 16 = acetate:succinate CoA transferase; 17 = succinate thiokinase; 18 = hydrogenase; 19 = adenylate kinase; 20 = H^+-driven ATPase (for details see Marvin-Sikkema *et al.*, 7,10).

for synthesis of ATP by way of reactions catalyzed by acetate:succinate CoA transferase and succinate thiokinase. At this stage it is unknown whether additional biologically useful energy is obtained in the hydrogenosome as a result of the net movement of protons and other ions. A polyclonal antibody directed against the C-terminal microbody protein targeting-signal SKL recognized a 30 kDa band and a 60 kDa band in whole cell-free extracts and in preparations of hydrogenosomes. These proteins are the subunits of the hydrogenosomal enzyme hydrogenase. The hydrogenase was purified to homogeneity. Full inhibition of the hydrogenase was obtained by CO, NO_2^- and acetylene, suggesting it could have been a (Ni-Fe-Se) type of hydrogenase, which would be the first indication of this type of enzyme in a eukaryote.

It is concluded that the hydrogenosome plays an important role in energy metabolism, maximizing the yield of biologically useful energy.

Introduction

Although recognized as late as 1975, the anaerobic zoosporic fungi or rumen fungi – as we will also call them in this paper, even though they are also found in the large intestines of both ruminant and non-ruminant herbivores – have drawn considerable attention. In the first place, they were the first strict anaerobic fungi to be discovered and no other groups of fungi have so far been described that complete their life cycle under completely anoxic conditions. Secondly, various studies have shown that in the herbivore gut the rumen fungi play an important quantitative role in the digestion of plant cell walls. Considerable emphasis has been given to the fact that the rumen fungi produce many exo-enzymes capable of hydrolyzing plant polymers of the plant cell wall, especially (hemi)celluloses. The specific activities of some of these enzymes (cellulase, xylanase) are the highest ever reported (see review by Wubah *et al.*, 17). This has led to some speculation regarding possible applications of the fungi or their enzymes in agriculture and industry.

On the basis of morphology the fungi were initially placed in the specially created family of the Neocallimasticaceae belonging to the order Spizellomycetales, which is one of the four orders in the class of Chytridiomycetes. This family has now been raised to the level of an order, the Neocallimasticales. So far, 16 species within 5 genera of anaerobic fungi have been described. Three genera (*Neocallimastix, Caecomyces, Piromyces*) develop a monocentric thallus, while the two other genera (*Orpinomyces, Ruminomyces* = *Anaeromyces*) are polycentric.

The life cycle of some anaerobic fungi has been studied. There is an alteration between a vegetative, sessile rhizoid stage which develops into a zoosporangium and a motile stage, the flagellated zoospore, released from the zoosporangium. No sexual stages have been described. As some authors have reported the successful isolation of rumen fungi from dried-out herbivore faeces and others reported the formation of a resistant stage in cultures, it has been proposed that there might be a third stage, *i.e.* an aero-tolerant survival stage in the form of a resistant sporangium or cyst, formed during desiccation of faeces (3). Living in an energy-limited environment, the rumen fungi must possess efficient mechanisms for harvesting biologically useful energy needed for the synthesis and excretion of the extracellular enzymes as well as for the completion of a 24-hr life cycle in order to prevent washout from the gut. It is known that energy is obtained by the fermentation of carbohydrates. Anaerobic fungi are able to grow on a large range of poly-, oligo-, and mono-saccharides. In pure culture the fungi eliminate more varied endproducts of carbohydrate catabolism than any other eukaryote studied. In axenic culture, most strains produce H_2, CO_2, formate, acetate, lactate and ethanol from carbohydrates, while in addition small amounts of succinate and malate are sometimes reported. As far as we know the production of formate is unique for eukaryotes. In the mixed microbial population, as a result of the transfer of hydrogen to hydrogen-oxidizing organisms (*e.g.* methanogenic bacteria: Bauchop and Mountfort, 1), the fungus strongly decreases its production of the other electron-sink products: lactate, ethanol and succinate. It has been shown that the activities of extracellular hydrolytic enzymes involved in polysaccharide degradation and the ratios in which these enzymes are produced may also be changed in methanogenic co-cultures. Whether this is caused by a lowered hydrogen pressure in the co-culture or whether these changes are an effect of the increased fungal growth rate in the presence of the methanogens remains to be established. Pathways used for glucose catabolism during growth have been proposed for two species of *Neocallimastix* by Yarlett *et al.* (18) and O'Fallon *et al.* (14). It was found that a special membrane-bound organelle, the hydrogenosome, is involved in the final stages of glucose catabolism. Hydrogenosomes are small organelles found in several groups of parasitic or free-living anaerobic protists. In all these eukaryotes the hydrogenosome contains enzymes for the oxidation of malate and/or pyruvate. In *N. patriciarum* (18) the oxidation of malate to acetate, H_2 and CO_2 was also found to be located in hydrogenosomes. Unexpectedly, O'Fallon *et al.* (14) reported that in another species (*N. frontalis*) one of the enzymes in this pathway, *i.e.* pyruvate:ferredoxin oxidoreductase was lacking. From these publications it is not clear whether and how the fungal hydrogenosome plays a role in energy transduction. In view of questions raised by the proposed metabolic schemes we decided to study in detail the energy metabolism of a strain of the genus *Neocallimastix* sp. L2 one of us (F.D. M-S.) isolated from llama faeces. The characteristics of this strain have been described (7). In view of the central role of hydrogen in the mixed culture, we especially wanted to obtain more insight in the role of hydrogenosomes in H_2-production and energy-generation in anaerobic fungi. In addition, we wanted to obtain clues as to the evolutionary origin of these organelles. This chapter reports on the main results of this work, which served as the basis for a PhD thesis (5), of which the principal results were published in a series of papers (6, 7, 8, 9, 10, 11).

Fungi and methanogens: the central role of molecular hydrogen

Initial experiments (6) confirmed previous observations by other authors that in two-membered co-cultures of various species of fungi with methanogenic bacteria, the latter convert the fungal products hydrogen and formate to methane. Under these conditions practically the only other fungal products are carbon dioxide and acetate. This confirmed earlier studies with methanogenic co-cultures. Since lactate and ethanol do not function as substrates for methanogens, the conclusion must be that the fungus shuts down the production of these products in an environment where the partial hydrogen pressure is low. From co-culture experiments with methanogens that do not use formate, but still cause the shift towards acetate and carbon dioxide at the expense of lactate, ethanol and succinate, it was concluded that removal of formate is not involved in this regulation (6). It is the concentration of dissolved hydrogen gas, therefore, which apparently plays a regulatory role. The signal for this regulatory mechanism is unknown. The remarkable changes in the specific activities of the fungal enzymes involved in the formation of succinate, lactate and ethanol is a result of co-cultivation with methanogens and parallels the observed shift in products (see below). We confirmed and extended the observations made by Bauchop and Mountfort (1) that both rate and extent of the fermentation of cellulose by the fungi as well as growth rate and yield of the fungi growing on cellulose were increased in methanogenic co-cultures (6). Our studies were done with the fungal strains *N. frontalis* RE1, *N. patriciarum* CX, our strain *N.* sp. L2, *Piromyces communis* P and *Caecomyces* (Sphaeromonas) *communis* FG10 in co-culture with either *Methanobacterium bryantii* OGC 110, *Methanobrevibacter smithii* PS or *Methanobrevibacter arboriphilus* strain AZ.

Pathway of glucose catabolism in *Neocallimastix* sp. L2

In order to detect the enzymes involved in the catabolism of glucose to the fermentation products observed in *Neocallimastix*, cell-free extracts (CFE), as well as cytosolic (CY) and hydrogenosomal (HY) fractions after fractionation and separation of a hydrogenosome-enriched pellet were analyzed for the presence of enzymes. The method developed for preparing HY is described in Marvin-Sikkema *et al.* (8).

A number of enzymes that can play a role in hexose catabolism in anaerobic microorganisms were never detected in cell-free extracts (CFE), nor in the cytosolic fraction freed from hydrogenosomes (CY), nor in hydrogenosomal pellets (HY). These enzymes not found include: glucose-6-P dehydrogenase, PP_i-dependent phosphofructokinase, pyruvate carboxylase, pyruvate decarboxylase, citrate synthase, citrate lyase, phosphotransacetylase, acetate kinase, formate dehydrogenase, formate hydrogen lyase, NADH- or NADPH-oxidase, NADH- or NADPH-peroxidase, catalase, and superoxide dismutase.

In the CFE as well as in the CY the enzymes hexokinase, ATP-dependent phosphofructokinase and enolase were present as well as all the enzymes required for the reactions leading from phosphoenolpyruvate (PEP) to acetylCoA plus formate, lactate, ethanol and succinate. In CFE and in HY, but not in CY all enzymes involved in the oxidation of malate to acetylCoA, carbon dioxide and hydrogen were detected. The HY fraction also contained an adenylate kinase activity and an ATPase, while indirect evidence was obtained for the presence of an ADP/ATP translocase at the hydrogenosomal membrane (see below).

From these enzyme measurements a scheme (Fig. 14.1) was proposed for a possible route of glucose catabolism. Glucose is catabolized to PEP via the Embden-Meyerhof-Parnas pathway. PEP is either converted to pyruvate or to malate in the cytosol. Pyruvate in the cytosol is either oxidized to acetylCoA and formate or reduced to lactate. AcetylCoA may be reduced to ethanol. Malate is the chief substrate for the hydrogenosomes, as was later proven with hydrogenosomal suspensions (see below). Pyruvate is an intermediate in the malate oxidation. The energy in acetylCoA is used for synthesis of ATP by way of the reactions catalyzed by acetate:succinate CoA transferase and succinate thiokinase. It seems likely that the acetylCoA from the cytosol is also channelled through the thiokinase reaction, but we have no clues as to how acetylCoA passes the hydrogenosomal membrane. Electrons from the oxidation of malate and pyruvate are transferred to protons via ferredoxin. Molecular hydrogen is finally formed during reoxidation of reduced ferredoxin catalyzed by a hydrogenase which was present in the HY in high levels. Of the enzymes needed to reduce pyruvate to lactate, acetaldehyde to ethanol and fumarate to succinate both a NADH and a NADPH-dependent form was present in the CY. Both a NAD- and a NADP-linked malic enzyme activity and both a NADH:ferredoxin oxidoreductase and an NADPH-dependent form of this enzyme were detected in the HY fraction. In the mixed culture of the normal rumen environment as well as in co-cultures with hydrogen-oxidizing bacteria, the chief flux of electrons is through the organelle, but in other situations where the hydrogen pressure is allowed to build up, or the hydrogenosome function is inhibited in some other way, reduced products are formed in the cytosol allowing reoxidation of reduced cofactors. This catabolic route is not only in accord with the pattern of endproducts formed by *Neocallimastix* sp. L2 in pure culture, but ^{13}C-NMR analysis of the supernatant of 1-^{13}C-glucose-grown cultures did show that the ^{13}-C-label was found only in acetate (C_2-carbon), lactate (C_3), succinate (C_2), and ethanol (C_2), confirming the proposed route.

Proof of the localization of enzymes in hydrogenosomes

Hydrogenosomes are found in the rhizoid mycelium in our strain of *Neocallimastix* sp. L2, where they have a microbody-like appearance, and in the zoospore, where they often look elongated and show long extensions towards the flagellar pole. The hydrogenosomes have internal structures and invaginations, which are not understood. The organelle is surrounded by a single membrane.

Enzyme activities in cell-free extracts prepared from mycelium and zoospores were compared and it was found that hydrogenosomal enzyme activities were 2- to 6-fold higher in zoospores, while levels of some cytosolic enzymes were of equal magnitude.

When the same amounts of protein from both mycelium and zoospores were subjected to SDS-polyacryamide gel-electrophoresis followed by western blotting with antibodies raised against purified hydrogenosomes, a comparison of the intensities of cross reacting bands of mycelium and zoospore proteins indicated that the zoosporic preparation contained higher levels of hydrogenosomal proteins.

Further evidence for the localization of certain enzymes in hydrogenosomes was obtained by the use of hydrogenosome-enriched pellets. Sucrose density centrifugation was applied to the HY fraction and the following enzyme activities were found to coincide at the same sucrose density as the purified hydrogenosomes: 'malic enzyme', pyruvate:ferredoxin oxidoreductase (PFOR), NAD(P):ferredoxin oxidoreductase, acetate:succinate CoA transferase, succinate thiokinase and hydrogenase.

When these enzyme activities were assayed using isolated hydrogenosomes in an osmotically stabilized system in the presence or absence of 0.1% Triton X-100, an increased activity with Triton was found for 'malic enzyme', adenylate kinase and NAD(P)H:ferredoxin oxidoreductase, suggesting that the hydrogenosomal membrane is a barrier towards the substrates for these enzymes. When pyruvate:ferredoxin oxidoreductase activities were compared in both systems, it was found that Triton X-100 itself was inhibitory to this enzyme.

Of great value was the use of a polyclonal antibody directed against the C-terminal microbody protein targeting-signal SKL (obtained from Dr.S. Subramani). In western blots the anti-SKL antibody recognized a 30 kDa band in CFE, which was also recognized in purified hydrogenosomal preparations and later also in the purified hydrogenase fraction together with a minor band of 60 kDa.

Further support for the hydrogenosomal localization of proteins containing the C-terminal SKL sequence was obtained by immunofluorescence and immunocytochemistry (see Marvin-Sikkema *et al.*, 9).

Malic enzyme did not react with the anti-SKL polyclonal antibody, but there may be multiple targeting signals in hydrogenosomal proteins just as is the case for peroxisomal and glycosomal proteins. At this moment we do not know whether the other enzymes detected in the hydrogenosome carry the SKL-terminus.

Characteristics of the fungal hydrogenase

The hydrogenase was purified by anion exchange chromatography and hydrophobic interaction chromatography. The native MW of the purified hydrogenase was 87 kDa as determined by gel filtration, while the MW of the subunits as determined with SDS-PAGE were 30 and 60 kDa. Further characterization of the nature of the hydrogenase was obtained from inhibition experiments which showed full inhibition of the hydrogenase by CO, NO_2^-, acetylene, suggesting it could have been a (Ni-Fe-Se) type of hydrogenase. If this were true, it would be the first indication of this type of enzyme in a eukaryote (5).

Experiments with hydrogenase inhibitors

In 7-day incubations of the fungus in the presence of the hydrogenase inhibitor metronidazole (30 µM) or in incubations under a gas phase consisting of the hydrogenase inhibitor CO, a significant reduction in the rate of glucose consumption with a switch towards the formation of less molecular hydrogen and more lactate was seen, demonstrating the plasticity of the organism's metabolism. Meanwhile, there was hardly any change in the specific activities of several hydrogenosomal and cytosolic enzymes as measured in CFE, except that the activity of hydrogenase was depressed by 90% in the case of metronidazole and by 60% in the incubations with CO (Fig. 14.2). In view of the long incubation times in the presence of inhibitors, short term effects and long term adaptations can not be separated and the observed effects may be a result of a mixture of both. For example, metronidazole is itself an electron sink competing for electrons with protons and the compound falls apart when reduced. Therefore, the fungi may not have

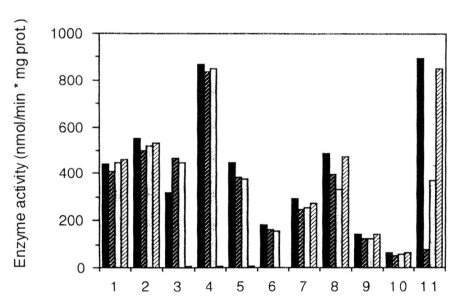

Figure 14.2. Enzyme activities in cell-free extracts from *Neocallimastix* sp. L2 cultured for 7 days in axenic culture in the absence of inhibitors (black columns), or in the presence of metronidazole (30 µM; dark-hatched bars), CO (20% v/v in the gas phase; grey columns), or in the presence of *Methanobrevibacter smithii* (light-hatched columns).

Enzyme activities measured: 1 = hexokinase; 2 = phosphofructokinase; 3 = lactate dehydrogenase; 4 = acetaldehyde dehydrogenase; 5 = alcohol dehydrogenase; 6 = fumarate reductase; 7 = malic enzyme; 8 = NADH:ferredoxin oxidoreductase; 9 = NADPH:ferredoxin oxidoreductase; 10 = pyruvate:ferredoxin oxidoreductase; 11 = hydrogenase (for details see ref. 9).

been exposed to sufficiently high levels of metronidazole to completely block hydrogenase function. Perhaps this is also the reason why it has not been possible to make fungi hydrogenase-free, even not after transferring the organism weekly for over 3 years to a metronidazole-containing culture medium. The inhibitor was only added to the fresh medium before inoculation, but metronidazole concentrations were not monitored during growth (10).

By way of comparison the dramatic changes seen in the activities of some enzymes of the fungus after growth in methanogenic co-cultures are also shown in Fig. 14.2. The enzymes fumarate reductase, lactate dehydrogenase, acetaldehyde dehydrogenase and alcohol dehydrogenase were down-regulated between 70- and 140-fold in the co-culture of *Neocallimastix* L2 and *Methanobrevibacter smithii* as compared to the fungal monoculture (Marvin-Sikkema *et al.*, 10), whereas specific activities of hexokinase, phosphofructokinase and, surprisingly, the specific activities of the hydrogenosomal enzymes remained practically unaltered.

Hydrogenosomes contain a novel ATP-ase

Further studies on HY (Marvin-Sikkema *et al.*, 11) revealed that the activity peak of hydrogenase, the marker enyzme of the hydrogenosomes, coincided with a peak of an ATPase at a sucrose density of 1.25–1.26 g. ml^{-1}. Fractions from the sucrose gradient with these densities were pooled for experiments to study the properties of the hydrogenosomal ATPase. The apparent K_m for ATP was 1.2 mM. The pH-optimum of the ATPase was pH 8.5 and Mg^{2+} or Mn^{2+}, but not Ca^{2+} or Co^{2+} were required.

It was ruled out that alkaline phosphatase or 5'-nucleotidase activity were causing the ATP-hydrolysis: both enzymes were absent from the HY, which is at the same time an indication that no contamination with plasma membranes had occurred in the preparation of HY. The presence of P^{1}P^5-di(adenosin-5'-) pentaphosphate, a specific inhibitor of adenylate kinase, did not influence ATPase activity. This inhibitor in a concentration of 100 μM completely blocked the hydrogenosomal adenylate kinase.

The ATPase activity is novel in the sense that none of the known ATPase-inhibitors (N,N'-dicyclohexylcarbodiimide = DCCD, oligomycin, azide, vanadate, bafilomycin A$_1$, nitrate) blocked its activity However, the ATPase was completely blocked in the presence of 2 μM diethylstilbestrol (DES). When the ATPase assay was carried out in the presence of compounds (bongkrekic acid, carboxyatractylate) known to inhibit ADP/ATP translocase, there was a fall in the ATPase of about 66% as compared to the inhibitor-free control measurements. However, the inhibitors had no effect on ATPase activity in the presence of 0.1% (v/v) Triton X-100. These data suggest that in addition to the presence of an unusual ATPase localized in the organelle, there probably is an ADP/ATP translocase associated with the organelle membrane (11).

The interior of hydrogenosomes is alkaline

From fluorescence microscope observations it was learned that hydrogenosomes contain an esterase which hydrolyzes the ester bond in the fluorescent pH-probe BCECF (2′,7′-bis-(2-carboxyethyl)-5 (and 6)-carboxyfluorescein). The isolated organelles retained the entrapped BCECF when stored on ice. Fluorescence measurements subsequently indicated that the interior of the organelle is alkaline vs. the outside medium which had a pH of 7.4. The $\triangle$pH could be abolished with the ATPase inhibitor DES. The results suggested that isolated hydrogenosomes were able to maintain a pH-gradient at the expense of residual ATP present in the intact organelle and that ATPase is involved in the generation of the $\triangle$pH (11).

No evidence could be obtained for the presence of an electron-gradient above the detection limit using the fluorescent probes oxonol VI and the lipophilic cation tetraphenylphosponium (11).

An assay for hydrogenosome function

Suspensions of intact hydrogenosomes in a medium osmotically stabilized with 250 mM sucrose, containing a K-HEPES-buffer of pH 7.4, succinate, MgATP or MgADP and malate as the electron-donating substrate, converted malate stoichiometrically to H_2, CO_2 and acetate under strictly anoxic conditions. There was no H_2-production from pyruvate, nor was pyruvate detected as a product excreted in the medium. The system could be used as an assay for hydrogenosome function by monitoring H_2-production (11).

Hydrogen production was strongly decreased when either succinate, MgATP or MgADP were omitted from the assay medium. Succinate is needed in catalytic amounts for the succinate thiokinase reaction. No hydrogen was evolved when 0.1% (v/v) Triton X-100 was present, when malate was absent or when pyruvate was substituted for malate.

Hydrogen production from malate was blocked completely after introduction of molecular oxygen. Some metabolic inhibitors that interfere with membrane function were also shown to affect hydrogenosome function. The ionophores valinomycin and/or nigericin and the protonophore CCCP drastically inhibited H_2-production. The ATPase inhibitor DES, but not the inhibitors previously found to have no effect on ATPase activity, strongly reduced H_2-production. The same is true for inhibitors of mitochondrial ADP/ATP translocase such as bongkrekic acid or carboxyatractylate which reduced H_2-production dramatically as well.

Discussion

Several theories exist concerning the function of hydrogenosomes in anaerobic eukaryotes. The organelles were thought to play a role in energy metabolism by Müller (12), while other authors (Lloyd and Coombs, 4) stressed the significance of hydrogenosomes in the protection of O_2-labile enzymes by O_2-scavenging enzymes. Indeed the enzyme NADH-oxidase was present in the sucrose gradient fraction that contained the hydrogenosomal enzymes.

It is certain that hydrogenosomes of anaerobic chytridiomycete fungi play a role in energy metabolism as they were found to function as compartments for the venting of reduced nucleotides in the form of hydrogen (18, 5), thus allowing more acetylCoA to be formed at the expense of hydrogen-sink products such as lactate, ethanol and succinate of which the formation is not linked to the formation of ATP. Per mole of hexose fermented 4 moles of ATP would be obtained when also the acetylCoA formed in the cytosol is channelled through the hydrogenosome, although the mechanism for the transport of acetylCoA remains a mystery at the moment.

The hydrogenosome will allow maximization of the yield of biologically useful energy, but only when the organism is growing under natural conditions with regard to its gaseous environment. In the mixed culture of the normal rumen environment as well as in co-cultures in the presence of hydrogen-oxidizing bacteria (low pH_2, high pCO_2), the chief flux of electrons is directed through the hydrogenosome, but in situations where the hydrogen pressure is allowed to build up, or where the function of the hydrogenosome is suppressed in some other way (hydrogenase inhibitors, low pCO_2), reduced products are formed in the cytosol allowing reoxidation of reduced cofactors. It is noteworthy that the levels of the enzymes fumarate reductase, lactate dehydrogenase, acetaldehyde dehydrogenase and alcohol dehydrogenase were strongly down-regulated in a co-culture of *Neocallimastix* L2 and *Methanobrevibacter smithii* as compared to the fungal monoculture, whereas specific activities of hexokinase, phosphofructokinase and, surprisingly, the specific activities of the hydrogenosomal enzymes remained practically unaltered. It must be concluded that even in the pure culture hydrogenosomal enzyme levels are fully expressed.

These results offer an explanation for the fact that both rate and extent of the fermentation of cellulose by these anaerobic fungi as well as growth rate and yield of the fungi growing on cellulose are increased in methanogenic co-cultures of the fungal strains. That this must be a general phenomenon was proven by the fact that in principle the same results were obtained with various chytridiomycete species belonging to the genera *Neocallimastix, Piromyces* and *Caecomyces*. The methanogenic partner may not be of great importance since a similar shift in fermentation products was obtained provided the methanogen consumed the hydrogen produced by the fungus. Formate transfer did not have a regulatory influence as it was not required for the observed shift in line with the cytosolic localization of its production. Consumption of protons in the formation of hydrogen would result in an alkalinization of the interior of the organelle. It is too early to tell whether the net movements of ions across the hydrogenosomal membrane do result in an extra gain of energy as a result of an increase of the proton-motive force. Experiments have to show which molecular species of malate and acetate are involved in transport across the hydrogenosomal membrane. It is not known also whether carbon dioxide or carbonate crosses the membrane. ATP synthesized in the reactions which involve acetate:succinate CoA transferase and succinate thiokinase can apparently be brought to the cytosol via exchange with ADP or ADP can be replenished via the adenylate kinase reaction. ATP can also be used to pump out protons in order to maintain the alkaline equilibrium.

Various hypotheses have been brought forward in explaining the origin of hydrogenosomes. These were *e.g.* discussed by Cavalier-Smith (2) and Müller (13): a) hydrogenosomes are derived from former eubacterial endosymbionts, b) hydrogenosomes are derived from mitochondria, and c) hydrogenosomes belong to the class of microbodies. Whatley *et al.* (15) suggested that hydrogenosomes of protozoa evolved from symbiotic clostridia. An argument in favour of the endosymbiont theory for the origin of hydrogenosomes is the similarity between the oxidation of pyruvate to acetate, hydrogen and carbon dioxide and clostridial pyruvate metabolism. The presence of the enzymes pyruvate:ferredoxin oxidoreductase and hydrogenase also points in that direction. In this respect it is remarkable that Wilson and Wood (16) discovered 'eubacterial traits' in the anaerobic fungus *Neocallimastix frontalis* as they stated that the cellulase of that species resembles that of *Clostridium thermocellum* in that the activity to crystalline cellulose resides in a multicomponent enzyme complex. Cavalier-Smith (2) thought it to be highly unlikely that the anaerobic chytridiomycete fungi would have acquired clostridia by phagocytosis and suggested that the fungi could have converted their peroxisomes into hydrogenosomes by the addition of peroxisomal transit sequences to cytosolic enzymes, which thus became hydrogenosomal enzymes. This matter is further discussed by Van der Giezen *et al.* in this book.

References

(1)   BAUCHOP, T. and MOUNTFORT, D.O. (1981). Cellulose fermentation by a rumen anaerobic fungus in both the absence and presence of rumen methanogens. Appl. Environ. Microbiol. 42: 1103–1110.

(2)   CAVALIER-SMITH, T. (1987). The simultaneous symbiotic origin of mitochondria, chloroplasts and microbodies. Ann. New York Acad. Sci. 503: 55–71.

(3)   DAVIES, D.R., THEODOROU, M.K., LAWRENCE, M.I.G. and TRINCI, A.P.J. (1993). Distribution of anaerobic fungi in the digestive tract of cattle and their survival in faeces. J. Gen. Microbiol. 139: 1395–1400.

(4)   LLOYD, D. and COOMBS, G.H. (1989). Aerotolerantly anaerobic protozoa: some unsolved problems, pp. 267–286. In (D. Lloyd, G.H. Coombs and T.A. Paget, eds.): Biochemistry and molecular biology of anaerobic protozoa. Harwood Academic Publishers, London.

(5)   MARVIN-SIKKEMA, F.D. 1993. Hydrogenosomes of the anaerobic fungus *Neocallimastix* sp. L2. Ph.D. Thesis. Haren, The Netherlands: University of Groningen, 123 pp.

(6)   MARVIN-SIKKEMA, F.D., RICHARDSON, A.J., STEW-

ART, C.S., GOTTSCHAL, J.C. and PRINS, R.A. (1990). Influence of hydrogen-consuming bacteria on cellulose degradation by anaerobic fungi. Appl. Environ. Microbiol. 56: 3793–3797.

(7) MARVIN-SIKKEMA, F.D., LAHPOR, G.A., KRAAK, M.N., GOTTSCHAL, J.C. and PRINS, R.A. (1992). Characterization of an anaerobic fungus from llama faeces. J. Gen. Microbiol. 138: 2235–2241.

(8) MARVIN-SIKKEMA, F.D., PEDRO GOMES, T.M., GRIVET, J-P., GOTTSCHAL, J.C. and PRINS, R.A. (1993). Characterization of hydrogenosomes and their role in glucose metabolism of *Neocallimastix* sp. L2. Arch. Microbiol. 160: 388–396.

(9) MARVIN-SIKKEMA, F.D., KRAAK, M.N., VEENHUIS, M., GOTTSCHAL, J.C. and PRINS, R.A. (1993). The hydrogenosomal enzyme hydrogenase from the anaerobic fungus *Neocallimastix* sp. L2 is recognized by antibodies, directed against the C-terminal microbody protein targeting signal SKL. Eur. J. Cell Biochem. 61: 86–91.

(10) MARVIN-SIKKEMA, F.D., REES, E., KRAAK, M.N., GOTTSCHAL, J.C. and PRINS, R.A. (1993). Influence of metronidazole, CO, CO_2, and methanogens on the fermentative metabolism of the anaerobic fungus *Neocallimastix* sp. L2. Appl. Environ. Microbiol. 59: 2678–2683.

(11) MARVIN-SIKKEMA, F.D., DRIESSEN, A.J.M., GOTTSCHAL, J.C. and PRINS, R.A. (1994). Metabolic energy generation in hydrogenosomes of the anaerobic fungus *Neocallimastix*: evidence for a functional relationship with mitochondria. Mycol. Res. 98, 205–212.

(12) MÜLLER, M. (1988). Energy metabolism of protozoa without mitochondria. Ann. Rev. Microbiol. 42: 465–488.

(13) MÜLLER, M. (1993). The hydrogenosome. J. Gen Microbiol. (in press).

(14) O'FALLON, J.V., WRIGHT, R.W. and CALZA, R.E. (1991). Glucose metabolic pathways in the rumen fungus *Neocallimastix frontalis* EB188. Biochem. J. 274: 595–599.

(15) WHATLEY, J.M., JOHN, P. and WHATLEY, F.R. 1979. From extracellular to intracellular: the establishment of mitochondria and chloroplasts. Proc. R. Soc. London Ser. B. 204: 165–187. (cited by Cavalier-Smith (2)).

(16) WILSON, C.A. and WOOD, T.M. (1992). Studies of the cellulase of the rumen anaerobic fungus *Neocallimastix frontalis*, with

special reference to the capacity to degrade crystalline cellulose. Enzyme Microbiol. Technol., 14: 258–264.

(17)   WUBAH, D.A., AKIN, D.E. and BORNEMAN, W.S. (1993). Biology, fiber-degradation and enzymology of anaerobic zoosporic fungi. Crit. Rev. Microbiol. 19: 99–115.

(18)   YARLETT, N., ORPIN, C.G., MUNN, E.A., YARLETT, N.C. and GREENWOOD, C.A. (1986). Hydrogenosomes in the rumen fungus *Neocallimastix patriciarum.* Biochem. J. 236: 729–739.

15

THE EVOLUTIONARY ORIGIN OF HYDROGENOSOMES FROM ANAEROBIC FUNGI

M. VAN DER GIEZEN, J.C. GOTTSCHAL and R.A. PRINS
Department of Microbiology, University of Groningen, P.O. Box 14, 9750 AA Haren, The Netherlands.

Summary

Hydrogenosomes are spherical organelles found in different eukaryotic organisms. Hydrogenosomes perform the conversion of pyruvate or malate to hydrogen and acetate, presumably with the concomitant production of ATP. The evolutionary origin of these fascinating organelles remains obscure. We propose a new way for endosymbiotic uptake of bacteria by fungi at their extreme hyphal tip. Three enzymes leading to the production of hydrogen: pyruvate:ferredoxin oxidoreductase, ferredoxin, and hydrogenase, which are usually encountered in prokaryotic anaerobes only, are found in hydrogenosomes. These factors have led us to propose that fungal hydrogenosomes arose by the endosymbiotic uptake of a eubacterium, probably of the clostridial type.

Introduction

Hydrogenosomes are spherical, membrane-surrounded organelles varying in diameter from 0.2 to 2 µm (24,18). They were first described by Lindmark and Müller (13) and are defined by their specialized biochemistry: under anoxic conditions they produce molecular hydrogen by oxidizing pyruvate or malate (27).

Hydrogenosomes are energy-generating organelles (21,42) which enable the organism to perform an oxidative metabolism following the initial glycolytic pathway.

Hydrogenosomes have been found in different anaerobic eukaryotic

195

organisms like parasitic protozoa (13,14), free-living ciliates (9), rumen ciliates (59,57), and anaerobic fungi (58,20).

In this review we will focus on the evolutionary origin of hydrogenosomes with particular emphasis on those from anaerobic fungi.

Metabolism and morphology

Anaerobic fungi can grow on a variety of structural carbohydrates present in forage fibre which they attack with a whole range of hydrolytic enzymes (39). Most strains produce H_2, CO_2, ethanol, acetate, lactate, and formate as major fermentation products (18).

Metabolic pathways during growth on glucose have been determined in *Neocallimastix patriciarum* (58), *Neocallimastix frontalis* EB188 (29), and *Neocallimastix* sp. L2 (21) recently identified as *N. frontalis* based on rRNA sequencing (unpublished data). In all three organisms initial sugar metabolism proceeds via the Embden-Meyerhof-Parnas pathway. Fig. 15.1 depicts the proposed schemes for glucose catabolism in *N.patriciarum* and *N. frontalis* L2. These pathways show strong resemblance to those encountered in Clostridia (10) and protozoa (2).

Hydrogenosomes in anaerobic fungi may have different appearances depending on the life-stage of the fungus. Anaerobic fungi have at least two different 'life stages': a vegetative rhizoid and a motile zoospore (18). Perhaps the survival structures seen by Milne *et al.* (22) represent a third life stage. Whether there exists yet another life stage in a different host as with *Callimastix cyclopis* (53) is not known and will probably be difficult to show.

In the vegetative rhizoid, hydrogenosomes appear as spherical bodies with an electron-dense matrix. In zoospores, however, hydrogenosomes have protrusions towards the flagellar pole (20). In anaerobic fungi hydrogenosomes are surrounded by a single membrane (20) and not by a double membrane as in parasitic protozoa (9).

Evolution of Eukaryotes

Before going into the details of the evolutionary origin of hydrogenosomes of anaerobic fungi some basic principles about eukaryotic evolution will be discussed.

In 1979 Whatley *et al.* (52) wrote: 'Evolutionary theories are necessarily more speculative than non-evolutionary theories since they deal

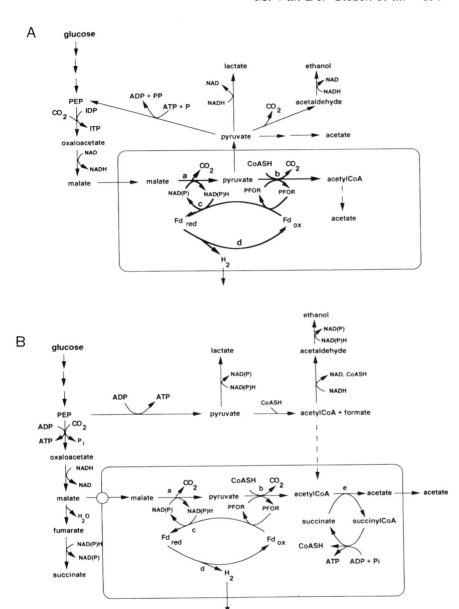

Figure 15.1. Glucose catabolic pathways of (A) *Neocallimastix patriciarum*, and (B) *Neocallimastix frontalis* L2. Reactions within box are associated with hydrogenosomes. a: 'malic enzyme'; b: pyruvate:ferredoxin oxidoreductase; c: NAD(P)H:ferredoxin oxidoreductase; d: hydrogenase; e: acetate:succinate CoA transferase.

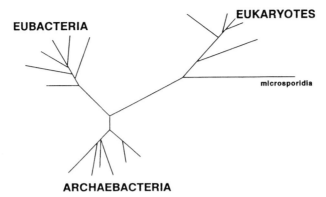

Figure 15.2. Phylogenetic tree of life based on small subunit rRNA sequences (Adapted from (55)).

with a complex series of events which happened over a long period, a long time ago'. This statement is reflected in the enormous amount of articles and existing theories about this subject.

The principle of biochemical evolution of macromolecules (54) gave a more or less objective basis for constructing a universal *arbor vitae*. Woese and his colleagues constructed such a tree as is depicted in Fig. 15.2, using nucleotide sequences of 16S and 18S rRNA (55). Because the nature of the oldest organism is not known the tree is not rooted. A generally accepted idea is that the last common ancestor can be found near the triple junction of the main branches. Different authors, using different arguments, urge for different junctions although most authors nowadays root the tree along the eubacterial branch (36). So, archaebacteria and eukaryotes are derived from a common ancestral eubacterium. Doolittle (8) argued that this branching happened relatively soon after the origin of life itself, probably at least 3.0 billion years ago while the oldest known microfossils date from 3.5 billion years ago.

So, how did the first eukaryotes originate in this relatively short time? Two major theories have been invented to explain the origin of eukaryotes, these are the autogenous origin hypothesis (32,41) and the endosymbiotic origin hypothesis (17). Most authors nowadays favour the symbiotic origin although using this scenario the nucleus is still supposed to be a product of an autogenous event. All cellular organelles like mitochondria and chloroplasts should have derived from bacteria which have been engulfed by the nucleate host. Cavalier-Smith (5) correctly stated that no bacteria can take up other living cells, so the nucleate host should have been something else. Most biologists are not aware of the fact that there exists an ancient group of eukaryotes (see Fig. 15.2, microsporidia) which are deficient of organelles (46,5,45). These Archezoa happen to be phagotrophic and could have been ideal candidates for taking up the endosymbionts (5).

By taking up cyanobacteria and purple nonsulfur bacteria, chloroplasts and mitochondria came into existence. The membranes of these organelles are not, like Schnepf stated (37), chimeric structures comprising the phagosome membrane and the bacterial plasma membrane but consist exclusively of bacterial membranes from the Gram-negative endosymbionts (5).

Peroxisomes should, in this view, originate from Gram-positive endosymbionts. The fact that peroxisomes do not, while mitochondria and chloroplasts do, contain any DNA is not in contradiction with this statement. Cavalier-Smith (4) argued that Gram-positives are more closely related to eukaryotes than Gram-negatives and so the host could probably provide most of the matrix proteins for the endosymbiont. Then, all the endosymbiont genes coding for such proteins could easily be lost. For membrane-proteins the insertion into the membrane would be relatively similar whether these came from the endosymbiont or from the cytoplasm of the host. There would thus be almost no barrier to the transfer of all the genes coding for membrane proteins into the nucleus. The metabolic efficiency of the organelles would be increased by the reduction of the volume occupied by DNA and ribosomes and this would be a selective advantage. So there should be no constraint for the complete loss of all the endosymbiont DNA when this endosymbiont was a Gram-positive bacterium.

The evolution of hydrogenosomes

As mentioned above, hydrogenosomes in protozoa are surrounded by a double membrane (and should therefore not be called microbodies as some authors do) whereas hydrogenosomes from anaerobic fungi are surrounded by a single membrane. Thinking of hydrogenosomes as endosymbionts, protozoan hydrogenosomes should therefore have come from Gram-negative bacteria because of their double membrane. But it could be possible that the outer membrane represents the phagosomal membrane as in the three-membraned chloroplasts from the Euglenoidea and Dinozoa (5). For these reasons hydrogenosomes from protozoa could originate from Gram-positive endosymbionts and because of the striking similarities with clostridial metabolism (see above) they could have been clostridial in nature (23,52).

A second possibility, gaining more and more support is that protozoan hydrogenosomes are degenerate mitochondria. Especially the findings that hydrogenosomal proteins contain a mitochondrion-like transit signal (11,12,3) seems to support this theory.

However, hydrogenosomes from anaerobic fungi do not contain proteins carrying mitochondrion-like signals. Recent findings of Marvin-Sikkema *et al.* (19) showed that a general microbody-targeting-signal is present on some hydrogenosomal proteins. Interestingly, Cavalier-Smith (5) argued that fungal hydrogenosomes originated from peroxisomes because it must be considered unlikely that fungi acquired Gram-positive endosymbionts by phagocytosis. He probably, implicitly, referred to the rigid cell wall of fungi and the fact that no phagocytosing fungi are known.

We think these conclusions are somewhat premature and we like to provide some food for thought by stressing that endosymbiosis could have happened in a different manner and possibly in a more recent period than often considered when discussing evolution of existing species.

Filamentous fungi grow by penetrating dead or living organic material with their hyphae. These hyphae grow by extension at their extreme tip. The cell wall of this growing tip is most plastic at the apex and becomes more rigid posteriorly. Extension of the hyphae is driven by turgor. Reinhardt (34) thought that the cell wall is extended by intussusception of wall material. But in the 1980's Wessels *et al.* (50) and Wessels (48) proposed a completely different theory which explained apical wall growth. This theory has been named the steady-state theory for apical wall growth. The term steady-state refers to the 'steady-state' quantity of plastic wall material at the tip of the hyphae.

This steady-state theory has been developed for ascomycetes and basidiomycetes but could also hold for other fungi possessing other wall polymers. The model is depicted in Fig. 15.3.

There appears to be some time between the enzymatic polymerization and the spontaneous crystallization of the chitin polymer chains (straight lines) (44), this is also the case for β-glucan (wavy lines) (38). Chitin forms microfibrils and β-glucan triple-helices which interact to form covalent linkages, but very little is known about the nature of these linkages (49).

At the extreme tip (A) the cell wall polymer chitin and β-glucan are deposited by apposition, these polymers are minimally cross-linked

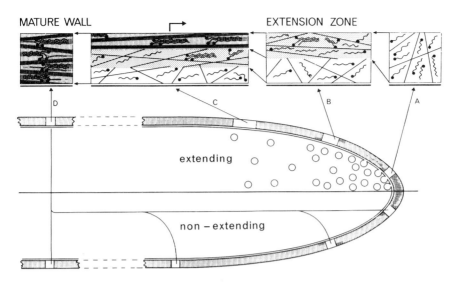

Figure 15.3. The steady-state model of apical wall growth. For the extending apex the schematic drawing represents the stretching of the wall and the addition of new wall material from the cytoplasmic side. Note that wall material moves from the inside to the outside and that the wall at the outside is always oldest. See text for explanation (from (51), reproduced with permission).

and so the cell wall is most plastic. Subapically (B) the newly added zone of cell wall polymers becomes stretched and the polymers form linkages while in the mean time new cell wall polymers are deposited at the apex. The stretching and cross-linking proceeds (increased shading) even further (C) until the cell wall is completely cross-linked (D). Areas with the same shading in (A), (B), and (C) represent equal volumes of hyphal wall. Because the extreme tip is most plastic, turgor pressure will expand this wall maximally and so the apposition site will be pushed away from the zone of rigidification which starts immediately behind the apex (51).

So, indeed, Cavalier-Smith has been right in pointing out the unlikelihood of phagocytosis by fungi through their rigid cell wall. But this may not hold for the extreme tip of growing hyphae!

Imagine a clostridial eubacterium which is squeezed between a solid substratum and an extending hyphae-tip. This bacterium could very well been completely engulfed by the extending tip. To become an endosymbiont the bacterium should also be taken up by the plasma membrane by endocytosis. Since endocytosis has been found to occur in *Saccharomyces cerevisiae* (16,35) and *Candida albicans* (1) this should probably be possible in other fungi as well. The only problem would have been to get rid of the fungal cell wall which encloses the newly formed endosymbiont. But this only needed to happen once during evolution because the new host would be so succesful that it would rapidly multiply and establish a new evolutionary branch.

The above scenario is not such an imaginary one as it might seem at first sight. For example, the symbiosis between *Rhizobium* and leguminous plants depends on a very similar event! When soil bacteria from the genus *Rhizobium* are in the neighbourhood of a root hair from a leguminous plant, the root hair starts to curl and the bacteria become entrapped. After local hydrolysis of the plant cell wall the bacteria enter the root cells by an invagination of the plasma membrane called the infection thread (15,28). This thread leads the bacteria to the root inner cortex where the already dividing bacteria form the nodule primordium (30). These primordia develop into mature root nodules in which the endosymbiontic bacteria fix molecular nitrogen. Although a lot is known about the root nodular formation still little is known about the exact processes of the endocytosis of bacteria in plant cells (43).

So, even though the plant cell wall and turgor pressure normally severely limit endocytosis (7) endosymbionts are created every day! Would it then be too unlikely to suppose that at some point in the evolution an (anaerobic) fungus took up a clostridial bacterium and enventually converted it into what we now call hydrogenosomes?

Conclusions

As mentioned above two theories exist to explain the origin of protozoan hydrogenosomes. In the first, which is favoured by Müller (23,25,26) it is assumed that clostridia have been adopted as endosymbionts. In favour of this theory is the striking similarity between hydrogenosomal metabolism and clostridial metabolism.

In the second theory hydrogenosomes are seen as degenerated mitochondria (9). Arguments in favour of this latter theory are based primarily on studies of the mitochondrion-like transit signals found in hydrogenosomal proteins (11,12,3). The presence of a double membrane can not be used as a decisive argument because of reasons mentioned above. A double membrane may originate from a mitochondrion or it could have come from a combination of the Gram-positive plasma membrane and the host phagosome membrane. Only detailed studies on the outer hydrogenosomal membrane will enable us to decide between these two possibilities.

Thus far no DNA has been detected in protozoan hydrogenosomes (40, 47) with the exception of the somewhat doubtful results reported by Čerkasovová *et al.* (6). The endosymbiont theory does not require DNA in Gram-positive endosymbionts because of the single membrane and the closer resemblance of Gram-positives and eukaryotes as discussed above (4). So we must conclude that at this moment most arguments are in favour for a clostridial origin for protozoan hydrogenosomes.

In the case of hydrogenosomes from anaerobic fungi the story is more or less the same. Because no double membrane is present on these hydrogenosomes a mitochondrial origin is unlikely because there is no case known were a Gram-negative bacterium has lost its outer membrane and its peptidoglycan layer (5).

The discovery of a general microbody targeting signal in hydrogenosomal proteins by Marvin-Sikkema *et al.* (19) favours a Gram-positive endosymbiont theory. The major question still open is whether the hydrogenosomes evolved from a clostridial endosymbiont or from peroxisomes.

Taking the set of enzymes in hydrogenosomes and comparing it with clostridial enzymes, a clostridial origin seems most likely. Especially pyruvate:ferredoxin oxidoreductase is a typical, ancient, clostridial enzyme. The hydrogenosomal metabolism which leads to the production of hydrogen is based on three enzymes: pyruvate:ferredoxin oxidoreductase, ferredoxin, and hydrogenase. This pathway is exceptional in eukaryotes but is present in numerous prokaryotic anaerobes (26). So, based on these arguments and on the hypothetical scenario mentioned above, we prefer the theory that fungal hydrogenosomes originated from a clostridial endosymbiont.

In order to find further support for a clostridial origin we are currently purifying the fungal hydrogenase as initiated by Marvin-Sikkema *et al.* (19) in order to isolate the genes coding for this essential hydrogenosomal protein. Sequence information of the hydrogenase genes will probably reveal the phylogenetic position of this protein relative to other known hydrogenase genes (33,31,56). Obtaining sequence information of other hydrogenosomal proteins, especially ferredoxin end pyruvate:ferredoxin oxidoreductase, will also be attempted in the near future.

A search for the presence of hydrogenosomal DNA will also be continued to reveal information on the evolutionary background of these fascinating organelles.

References

(1)   BASRAI, M.A., NAIDER, F. and BECKER, J.M. (1990). Internalization of lucifer yellow in *Candida albicans* by fluid-phase endocytosis. J.Gen.Microbiol. 136, 1059–1065.

(2)   BAUCHOP, T. (1971). Mechanism of hydrogen formation in *Trichomonas foetus*. J.Gen.Microbiol. 68, 27–33.

(3)   BRUL, S., KELTMAN, R.H., LOMBARDO, M.C.P. and VOGELS, G.D. (1994). Molecular cloning of hydrogenosomal ferredoxin cDNA from the anaerobic amoeboflagellate *Psalteromonas lanterna*. Biochim. Biophys. Acta 1183, 544–546.

(4)   CAVALIER-SMITH, T. (1987). The origin of eukaryote and archaebacterial cells. Ann. NY. Acad. Sci. 503, 17–54.

(5)   CAVALIER-SMITH, T. (1987). The simultaneous symbiotic origin of mitochondria, chloroplasts, and microbodies. Ann. NY. Acad. Sci. 503, 55–71.

(6)   ČERKASOVOVÁ, A., ČERKASOV, J., KULDA, J. and REISCHIG, J. (1976). Circular DNA and cardiolipin in hydrogenosomes, microbody-like organelles in *Trichomonas*. Folia Parasitol. 23, 33–37.

(7)   CRAM, W.J. (1980). Pinocytosis in plants. New Phytol. 84, 1–17.

(8)   DOOLITTLE, W.F. (1980). Revolutionary concepts in evolutionary cell biology. TIBS June, 146–149.

(9)   FINLAY, B.J. and FENCHEL, T. (1989). Hydrogenosomes in some anaerobic protozoa resemble mitochondria. FEMS Microbiol. Lett. 65, 311–314.

(10)   GRAY, C.T. and GEST, H. (1965). Biological formation of molecular hydrogen. Science 148, 186–192.

(11)   JOHNSON, P.J., D'OLIVEIRA, C.E., GORRELL, T.E. and MÜLLER, M. (1990). Molecular analysis of the hydrogenosomal ferredoxin of the anaerobic protist *Trichomonas vaginalis*. Proc. Natl. Acad. Sci. USA 87, 6097–6101.

(12)   LAHTI, C.J., D'OLIVEIRA, C.E. and JOHNSON, P.J. (1992). β-succinyl-coenzyme A synthetase from *Trichomonas vaginalis* is a soluble hydrogenosomal protein with an amino-terminal sequence that resembles mitochondrial presequences. J. Bacteriol. 174, 6822–6830.

(13)   LINDMARK, D.G. and MÜLLER, M. (1973). Hydrogenosome, a cytoplasmic organelle of the anaerobic flagellate *Tritrichomonas foetus*, and its role in pyruvate metabolism. J. Biol. Chem. 248, 7724–7728.

(14) LINDMARK, D.G., MÜLLER, M. and SHIO, H. (1975). Hydrogenosomes in *Trichomonas vaginalis*. J. Parasitol. 63, 552–554.

(15) LONG, S.R. (1989). Rhizobium-legume nodulation: life together in the underground. Cell 56, 203–214.

(16) MAKAROW, M. (1985). Endocytosis in *Saccharomyces cerevisiae*: internalization of α-amylase and fluorescent dextran into cells. EMBO J. 4, 1861–1866.

(17) MARGULIS, L. (1970). Origin of eukaryotic cells. Yale University Press, New Haven.

(18) MARVIN-SIKKEMA, F.D. (1993). Hydrogenosomes of the anaerobic fungus *Neocallimastix* sp. L2. Ph.D. Thesis. Haren, The Netherlands: University of Groningen.

(19) MARVIN-SIKKEMA, F.D., KRAAK, M.N., VEENHUIS, M., GOTTSCHAL, J.C. and PRINS, R.A. (1993). The hydrogenosomal enzyme hydrogenase from the anaerobic fungus *Neocallimastix* sp. L2 is recognized by antibodies, directed against the C-terminal microbody protein targetting signal SKL. Eur. J. Cell Biol. 61, 86–91.

(20) MARVIN-SIKKEMA, F.D., LAHPOR, G.A., KRAAK, M.N., GOTTSCHAL, J.C. and PRINS, R.A. (1992). Characterization of an anaerobic fungus from llama faeces. J. Gen. Microbiol. 138, 2235–2241.

(21) MARVIN-SIKKEMA, F.D., PEDRO-GOMES, T.M., GRIVET, J.-P., GOTTSCHAL, J.C. and PRINS, R.A. (1993). Characterization of hydrogenosomes and their role in glucose metabolism of *Neocallimastix* sp. L2. Arch.Microbiol. 160, 388–396.

(22) MILNE, A., THEODOROU, M.K., JORDAN, M.G.C., KING-SPOONER, C. and TRINCI, A.P.J. (1989). Survival of Anaerobic Fungi in Feces, in Saliva, and in Pure Culture. Exp. Mycol. 13, 27–37.

(23) MÜLLER, M. (1975). Biochemistry of protozoan microbodies: peroxisomes, α-glycerophosphate oxidase bodies, hydrogenosomes. Ann.Rev.Microbiol. 29, 467–483.

(24) MÜLLER, M. (1980). The hydrogenosome. In: The Eukaryotic Microbial Cell, 30th Symposium of the Society for General Microbiology, University of Cambridge. (Gooday, G.W., Lloyd, D. and Trinci, A.P.J. eds.) pp. 127–142. Cambridge University Press, London.

(25)   MÜLLER, M. (1987). Hydrogenosomes of trichomonad flagellates. Acta Universitatis Carolinae – Biologica 30, 249–260.

(26)   MÜLLER, M. (1988). Energy metabolism of protozoa without mitochondria. Ann. Rev. Microbiol. 42, 465–488.

(27)   MÜLLER, M. (1993). The hydrogenosome. J.Gen.Microbiol. 139, 2879–2889.

(28)   NAP, J.-P. and BISSELING, T. (1990). Developmental biology of a plant-prokaryote symbiosis: the legume root nodule. Science 250, 948–954.

(29)   O'FALLON, J.V., WRIGHT, R.W. and CALZA, R.E. (1991). Glucose metabolic pathways in the anaerobic rumen fungus *Neocallimastix frontalis* EB188. Biochem. J. 274, 595–599.

(30)   PICHON, M., JOURNET, E.-P., DEDIEU, A., DE BILLY, F., TRUCHET, G. and BARKER, D.G. (1992). *Rhizobium meliloti* elicits transient expression of the early nodulin gene ENOD12 in the differentiating root epidermis of transgenic alfalfa. Plant Cell 4, 1199–1211.

(31)   PRZYBYLA, A.E., ROBBINS, J., MENON, N.K. and PECK Jr., H.D. (1992). Structure-function relationships among the nickel-containing hydrogenases. FEMS Microbiol. Rev. 88, 109–136.

(32)   RAFF, R.A. and MAHLER, H.R. (1972). The non symbiotic origin of mitochondria; the question of the origin of the eucaryotic cell and its organelles reexamined. Science 177, 575–582.

(33)   REEVE, J.N. and BECKER, G.S. (1990). Conservation of primary structure in prokaryotic hydrogenases. FEMS Microbiol. Rev. 87, 419–424.

(34)   REINHARDT, M.O. (1892). Das Wachstum der Pilzhyphen. Jahrb. Wiss. Bot. 23, 479–565.

(35)   RIEZMAN, H. (1985). Endocytosis in yeast. Several of the yeast secretory mutants are defective in endocytosis. Cell 40, 1001–1009.

(36)   RUNNEGAR, B.N. (1992). The tree of life. In: The proterozoic biosphere; a multidisciplinary study. (Schopf, J.W. and Klein, C. eds.) pp. 471–475. Cambridge University Press, Cambridge.

(37)   SCHNEPF, E. (1964). Zur Feinstruktur von Geosiphon pyriforme; Ein Versuch zur Deutung cytoplasmatischer Membranen und Kompartimente. Arch. Mikrobiol. 49, 112–131.

(38)   SONNENBERG, A.S.M., SIETSMA, J.H. and WESSELS, J.G.H. (1985). Spatial and temporal differences in the synthesis

of (13)-β and (16)-β linkages in a wall glucan of *Schizophyllum commune*. Exp. Mycol. 9, 141–148.

(39) TEUNISSEN, M.J. and OP DEN CAMP, H.J.M. (1993). Anaerobic fungi and their cellulolytic and xylanolytic enzymes. Antonie Leeuwenhoek Int. J. Gen. Mol. Microbiol. 63: 63–76.

(40) TURNER, G. and MÜLLER, M. (1983). Failure to Detect Extranuclear DNA in *Trichomonas vaginalis* and *Tritrichomonas foetus*. J. Parasitol. 69(1), 234–236.

(41) UZZELL, T. and SPOLSKY, C. (1974). Am. Sci. 62, 334.

(42) VAN DER GIEZEN, M., MARVIN-SIKKEMA, F.D., GOTTSCHAL, J.C. and PRINS, R.A. (1993). Hydrogenosomes of the anaerobic fungus *Neocallimastix* sp. L2. In: Metabolic Compartmentation in Yeasts; Abstracts of the Sixteenth International Symposium on Yeasts (ISSY16); Arnhem, The Netherlands; August 23–26, 1993. (Scheffers, W.A. and van Dijken, J.P. eds.) pp. 304–308.

(43) VERMA, D.P.S. (1992). Signals in root nodule organogenesis and endocytosis of *Rhizobium*. Plant Cell 4, 373–382.

(44) VERMEULEN, C.A. and WESSELS, J.G.H. (1986). Chitin biosynthesis by a fungal membrane preparation. Evidence for a transient non-crystalline state of chitin. Eur. J. Biochem. 158, 411–415.

(45) VOSSBRINCK, C.R., MADDOX, T.J., FRIEDMAN, S., DE-BRUNNER-VOSSBRINCK, B.A. and WOESE, C.R. (1987). Ribosomal RNA sequence suggests microsporidia are extremely ancient eukaryotes. Nature 326, 411–414.

(46) VOSSBRINCK, C.R. and WOESE, C.R. (1986). Eukaryotic ribosomes that lack a 5.8S RNA. Nature 320, 287–288.

(47) WANG, A.L. and WANG, C.C. (1985). Isolation and characterization of DNA from *Tritrichomonas foetus* and *Trichomonas vaginalis*. Mol. Biochem. Parasitol. 14, 323–335.

(48) WESSELS, J.G.H. (1986). Cell wall synthesis in apical hyphal growth. Int. Rev. Cytol. 104, 37–79.

(49) WESSELS, J.G.H. (1990). Role of wall architecture in fungal tip growth generation. In: Tip growth in plant and fungal cells. (Heath, I.B. ed.) pp. 1–29. Academic Press, San Diego.

(50) WESSELS, J.G.H., SIETSMA, J.H. and SONNENBERG, A.S.M. (1983). Wall synthesis and assembly during hyphal morphogenesis in *Schizophyllum commune*. J. Gen. Microbiol. 129, 1599–1605.

(51) WESSELS, J.G.H. (1993). Tansley review no. 45; Wall growth,

protein excretion and morphogenesis in fungi. New Phytol. 123, 397–413.

(52)   WHATLEY, J.M., JOHN, P. and WHATLEY, F.R. (1979). From extracellular to intracellular: the establishment of mitochondria and chloroplasts. Proc. R. Soc. Lond. B 204, 165–187.

(53)   WHISLER, H.C., ZEBOLD, S.L. and SHEMANCHUK, J.A. (1975). Life History of *Coelomomyces psorophorae*. Proc. Natl. Acad. Sci. USA 72, 693–696.

(54)   WILSON, A.C., CARLSON, S.S. and WHITE, T.J. (1977). Biochemical evolution. Ann. Rev. Biochem. 46, 573–639.

(55)   WOESE, C.R. (1987). Bacterial Evolution. Microbiol.Rev. 51, 221–271.

(56)   WU, L.-F. and MANDRAND, M.A. (1993). Microbial hydrogenases: Primary structure, classification, signatures and phylogeny. FEMS Microbiol. Rev. 104, 243–270.

(57)   YARLETT, N., HANN, A.C., LLOYD, D. and WILLIAMS, A.G. (1983). Hydrogenosomes in a mixed isolate of *Isotricha prostoma* and *Isotricha intestinalis* from ovine rumen contents. Comp. Biochem. Physiol. 74B, 357–364.

(58)   YARLETT, N., ORPIN, C.G., MUNN, E.A., YARLETT, N.C. and GREENWOOD, C.A. (1986). Hydrogenosomes in the rumen fungus *Neocallimastix patriciarum*. Biochem. J. 236, 729–739.

(59)   YARLETT, N., HANN, A.C., LLOYD, D. and WILLIAMS, A.G. (1981). Hydrogenosomes in the rumen protozoon *Dasytricha ruminantium* Schuberg. Biochem. J. 200, 365–372.

16

HYDROGENOSOMES; UBIQUITOUS ORGANELLES IN ANAEROBIC PROTOZOA AND ANAEROBIC FUNGI

S. BRUL[#], A. LAUWERS and G.D. VOGELS
Department of Microbiology and Evolutionary Biology, University of Nijmegen, Toernooiveld 6525 ED Nijmegen, The Netherlands

[#]Present address Unilever Research Laboratory, Research and Engineering Division, Section Microbiology & Hygenic Processing, Olivier van Noortlaan 120, NL. 3133 AT Vlaardingen, The Netherlands

Summary

Hydrogenosomes are organelles which are often present in anaerobic protozoa (parasitic/free-living) and anaerobic rumen fungi. Despite their ubiquitous occurrence, not much is known as yet on their cellular functions, biogenesis and origin. In this review hydrogenosomes from protozoa and fungi will be compared with regard to key aspects of their morphology, function and protein targeting mechanisms. Recent literature data are reviewed together with some further molecular information of our laboratory on hydrogenosomes in a free-living anaerobic protozoan. We conclude that hydrogenosomes probably are polyphyletic. With the outcome we will speculate on the relationship between hydrogenosomes and other organelles.

Introduction

Hydrogenosomes are characteristic organelles of anaerobic eukaryotic cells such as anaerobic protozoa and anaerobic rumen fungi. The organelles derive their name from the fact that they contain the enzyme hydrogenase and thus can produce molecular hydrogen using pyruvate or malate as substrate.

Often, the hydrogen is consumed by epi- or endosymbiotic methanogenic bacteria (discussed among others in Ref. 6). Here we will give a concise review of the most important characteristics of hydrogenosomes. The significance of major differences of hydrogenosomes in protozoa and fungi, respectively, will be discussed in the frame work of the evolutionary relation between hydrogenosomes and other cellular organelles (see also Refs 6,23).

Characteristics and metabolism

Hydrogenosomes were discovered in the early seventies in anaerobic parasitic protozoa (*Tritrichomonas foetus* and *Trichomonas vaginalis*) by Müller and coworkers [16,17]. In a density gradient the organelles can be retrieved at an equilibrium density of 1,22–1,26 g/cm^3 [16,17,20 and Voncken, F & Brul, S unpublished observations].

A schematic summary of our current knowledge of the metabolic pathways involved in glucose fermentation via the hydrogenosomes in the parasitic anaerobic protozoan *T. vaginalis* and the anaerobic fungus *Neocallimastix* sp. L2 is given in Figure 16.1. Mainly on morphological grounds, hydrogenosomes were classified as microbodies, a group of single membrane bounded organelles to which peroxisomes, glyoxysomes and glycosomes belong. Studies by Benchimol & de Souza [1] and Honigberg *et al.* [9] in *T. vaginalis* and *T. foetus* revealed, however, two closely apposed unit membranes around their hydrogenosomes. Zwart *et al.* [31] were the first to demonstrate hydrogenosomes in anaerobic free-living protozoa. By using a cytochemical staining, the presence of the enzyme hydrogenase was established. Also in this type of anaerobic protozoa the hydrogenosomes were surrounded by a double membrane. Considering additionally the fact that the hydrogenosomal metabolism is completely different from the metabolism of other microbodies, their microbody nature in trichomonads and free-living protozoa became more and more questionable during the last decade. In fact, for anaerobic protozoa the initial classification should most likely nowadays be considered as incorrect (see also paragraph **5. BIOGENESIS**). Pyruvate produced during glycolysis is, at least in *T. vaginalis*, considered to be the compound which is taken up by the hydrogenosomes and is then converted by the organelles into H_2, CO_2 and acetate (Figure 16.1).

Anaerobic fungi were also shown to contain hydrogenosomes. In contrast to the situation in protozoa, hydrogenosomes of anaerobic fungi are surrounded by only one unit membrane [20]. Yarlett *et al.* [30]

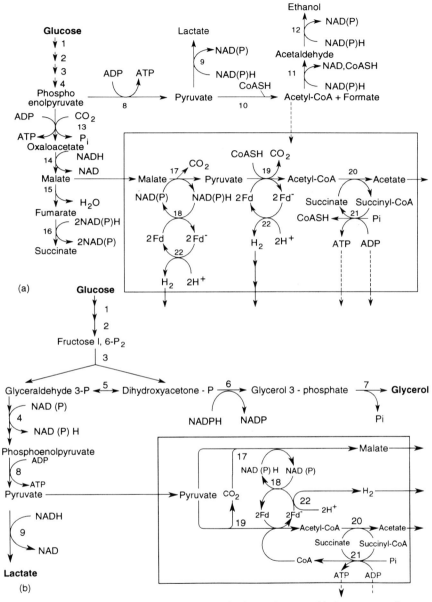

Figure 16.1. Metabolic routes of glucose fermentation in (a) the anaerobic fungus *Neocallimastix* sp. L2 [20] and (b) the anaerobic parasitic flagellate *Trichomonas vaginalis* [26] (Combined slightly modified figure taken with permission from Ref. 6). The boxed pathways are considered to be located in the hydrogenosomes. 1: hexokinase; 2: phosphofructokinase; 3: aldolase; 4: enolase; 5: triose phosphate isomerase; 6: glycerol 3-phosphate dehydrogenase (NADP); 7: glycerol 3-phosphatase; 8: pyruvate kinase; 9: lactate dehydrogenase; 10: pyruvate formate lyase ; 11: acetaldehyde dehydrogenase; 12: alcohol dehydrogenase; 13: phosphoenolpyruvate carboxy-lase/carboxykinase; 14: malate dehydrogenase ; 15: fumarase; 16: fumarate reductase ; 17:'malic enzyme'; 18: NAD(P)H:ferredoxin oxidoreductase 19: pyruvate:ferredoxin oxidoreductase; 20: acetate:succinate CoA transferase; 21: succinate thiokinase; 22: hydrogenase. Glucose fermentation via the hydrogenosomes yields 2 ATP in *Neocallimastix* sp. L2. In the parasite *Trichomonas vaginalis*, understrictly anaerobic conditions, only one extra ATP is synthesized per fermented glucose molecule (see text).

were the first to report on the biochemistry of the hydrogenosomes in these organisms. Their scheme on the metabolism of the organelles in *Neocallimastix* sp. was recently extended by studies of Marvin-Sikkema *et al.* [20]. At least the major part of the cytosolically produced pyruvate is thought to be converted into malate before transport over the membrane occurs. Acetate and molecular hydrogen are produced from the incorporated malate. Other end products of the metabolism of anaerobic fungi are ethanol, formate and lactate. These are, however, produced in the cytosol (Figure 16.1).

An important consequence of the fact that the fungal hydrogenosomes take up malate and not, as do *T. vaginalis* hydrogenosomes, pyruvate is that under strictly anaerobic conditions the net yield of glucose fermentation through the hydrogenosomal pathway is two high energy phosphate bonds. In contrast, this metabolic route leads to an overall synthesis of only one high energy phosphate bond in *T. vaginalis*. This is caused by the fact that in order to maintain the cytosolic redox balance, hydrogenosomal pyruvate to acetate conversion has to be accompanied by cytosolic glycerol phosphate breakdown and thus leads ultimately to the waste of one ATP.

Knowledge of the hydrogenosomal metabolism of anaerobic free-living protozoa awaits purification of the organelles from these organisms. This has been hampered by the fact that axenic mass cultivation of anaerobic free-living protozoa has not yet been achieved. However, measurements on whole cells have shown for monoxenic cultures of the anaerobic free-living ciliate *Trimyema compressum* that acetate, lactate, ethanol, formate, succinate, CO_2 and H_2 are metabolic end products of the organism [7]. From these observations one might infer a '*Neocallimastix* type' of glucose fermentation in this free-living anaerobic protozoan.

Function

In anaerobic parasitic protozoa and anaerobic fungi the hydrogenosomes actually produce ATP during the oxidative decarboxylation of pyruvate (see Figure 16.1). In this respect the organelles form the anaerobic equivalent of mitochondria. In the proces of ATP generation the enzyme succinate thiokinase (STK) plays an important role. The genes coding for both the α- and β-subunit of STK, adenylate kinase (ADK) and the hydrogenosomal electron carrier ferredoxin (fd) have recently been cloned from the parasitic anaerobic flagellate *T. vaginalis*

Table 16.1 MOLECULAR WEIGHTS OF PCR PRODUCTS OF GENES CODING FOR HYDROGENOSOMAL PROTEINS.

ENZYME	PCR products; approximate molecular weights			
	T. vaginalis		P. lanterna	
	cDNA	gDNA	cDNA	gDNA
STK	600	600	600	ND
ADK	300	300	300	300
fd	250	250	230	230

Comparison of the molecular weights (bp) of PCR products, using cDNA or gDNA as template, of analogous parts of succinate thiokinase (STK), adenylate kinase (ADK) and the electron carrier ferredoxin (fd) of the anaerobic parasitic protozoan *T. vaginalis* and the anaerobic free-living protozoan *P. lanterna*. ND: not determined.

[10, 12–14]. These are the first hydrogenosomal proteins of which the DNA and protein sequence is known and were shown to be homologous to their mitochondrial counterparts. For all an N-terminal topogenic signal is predicted (see paragraph **5. BIOGENESIS**).

Until now no hydrogenosomes could be isolated from any free-living protozoan their exact hydrogenosomal metabolic routes are not known. However, molecular biological experiments using degenerate primers suggest, together with the already mentioned localisation of hydrogenase, that in the anaerobic free-living protozoan *Psalteriomonas lanterna* [2], similar proteins and hence we infer similar metabolic routes as identified in trichomonads are operative. We therefore presume that also in these cells hydrogenosomes contribute significantly to the cellular ATP level. Table 16.1 shows results of a typical PCR experiment.

For the β-subunit of STK, fd and ADK specific products with a similar molecular weight were amplified in reactions with *T. vaginalis* cDNA/gDNA and *P. lanterna* cDNA/gDNA. In addition cross-hybridization experiments indicate that the *T. vaginalis* and *P. lanterna* PCR products are homologous (Brul, S, unpublished observations). The *P. lanterna* PCR products were sequenced and used in the screening of a cDNA library of the anaerobic free-living protozoan. First results for *P. lanterna* ferredoxin indicate that the cDNA predicted protein sequence shows the highest homology with *T. vaginalis* ferredoxin; 23% identity and 32% conservative substitutions (amino acid polarity and charge, 47% if only polarity is considered) in a 100 amino acid overlap [5]. Bacterial expression of the cDNA upon cloning into a plasmid vector, resulted in a fusion protein of ferredoxin and the lac Z′ part of bacterial β-galactosidase. Using an antibody against the lac Z′

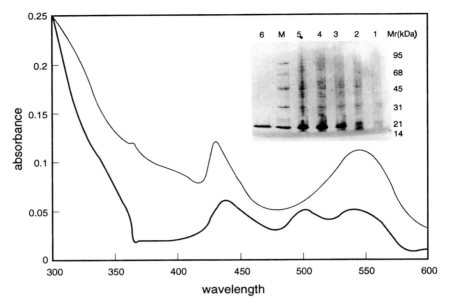

Figure 16.2. Absorption spectrum of the *Psalteriomonas lanterna* ferredoxin-*Escherichia coli* lac Z' fusion protein before (upper line) and after (lower line) reduction with sodium dithionite. Insert: 10–15% SDS polyacrylamide gelelectrophoresis of bacterial extracts 0–4 hours after induction of the ferredoxin-lac Z' protein (lanes 1–5) and of the purified fusion protein (lane 6). Purification was performed batchwise with anti β-galactosidase monoclonal antibodies according to a standard method used e.g. by Pharmacia-Biotech in their recombinant phage antibody system.

moiety, the fusion protein was purified to homogeneity (insert Figure 16.2). The absorption spectrum of the fusion protein showed typical characteristics of [2Fe-2S] centers alike the ones found in hydrogenosomal *T. vaginalis* ferredoxin with maxima at 360nm, 435nm and 550nm (Figure 16.2 cf. Ref. 19).

Upon reduction of the sample with sodium dithionite the 435nm peak became less than 40% of the native protein. Judging from the molar extinction coefficient at 435nm (cf. 458m, in Ref. 19) about 60% of the fusion protein contains the iron-sulfur cluster. Thus, as expected from the DNA sequence data, this preliminary information on the biochemistry of *P. lanterna* ferredoxin suggests that the proteins from this protozoan and *T. vaginalis* are indeed structurally and functionally homologous.

Recently Marvin-Sikkema *et al.* [22] demonstrated that, in contrast to the situation in trichomonads [18], in anaerobic fungi a hydrogenosomal ATPase is present which generates the observed proton motive force (pmf) over the hydrogenosomal membrane (hydrogenosomal lumen alkaline). This pmf could be used for e.g. the transport of substrates over the hydrogenosomal membrane or may be necessary for hydrogenosome biogenesis. Alternatively, the proton gradient may be generated through an as yet unknown mechanism involving a membrane bound electron transport chain, associated oxidation/reduction reactions, and scalar and vectorial H^+ translocation over the hydrogenosomal membrane. The proton gradient could subsequently drive the generation of (extra) ATP mediated by the membrane bound ATP-ase which would then function in the reverse direction as an ATP-synthase. Whatever will turn out to be true, incubating hydrogenosomes of *Neocallimastix* sp. with dissipators of a membrane proton gradient results in a strong impairment of H_2 production upon malate addition. Thus normal hydrogenosomal function in fungi depends on the presence of a membrane proton gradient [22].

Biogenesis

Hydrogenosomes are presumed to multiplicate through growth and division of preexisting organelles, essentially analogous to mitochondria and microbodies [3,25]. In *T. vaginalis* Lahti & Johnson [12] showed that hydrogenosomal proteins are synthesized in the cytosol on free ribosomes. Thus, a post-translational import of these proteins was invoked. Johnson *et al.* [10] showed for hydrogenosomal ferredoxin of *T. vaginalis* that a difference exists between the cDNA derived protein sequence and the actual protein sequence after purification from cellular homogenates. N-terminally eight extra amino acids were codified. A similar observation was made for the *T. vaginalis* hydrogenosomal α- and β-subunit of STK [13,14], ADK [15] and a similar situation was inferred for *P. lanterna* fd [5]. Helical wheel projections showed that the N-terminal sequences might contain topogenic information in the form of an amphiphilic α-helix. In this respect, the organelles appear to be similar to mitochondria where most proteins contain an N-terminal topogenic signal sequence. Most microbody proteins on the other hand contain a C-terminal non cleavable signal sequence which consists of the tripeptide serine-lysine-leucine (SKL) [8]. In immunological experiments using a specific anti-(C-terminal)SKL antiserum Keller *et al.* [11] observed no cross-reactivity with *T. vaginalis* hydrogenosomes.

In contrast, Marvin-Sikkema *et al.* [21] recently did observe a cross-reaction of the anti-(C-terminal) SKL antiserum with *Neocallimastix* sp. L2 hydrogenosomes. After further characterization one of the main enzymes involved in this reaction turned out to be hydrogenase. Hence, hydrogenosomes of anaerobic fungi appear to differ also in this aspect from those of anaerobic (parasitic) protozoa and look more 'microbody-like'.

A definitive assessment of the topogenic mechanisms used by hydrogenosomal proteins in the various organisms awaits the development of reliable *in vitro* import systems and/or transformation protocols for anaerobic fungi and protozoa. A complementary experimental approach consists in expressing putative hydrogenosomal targeting sequences attached to passenger proteins in various yeasts and subsequently studying their effectiveness in mitochondrial or peroxisomal targeting. In this way information would be obtained concerning the question whether hydrogenosomal (putative) targeting sequences are functionally equivalent to either microbody or mitochondrial topogenic sequences.

Evoluationary origins of hydrogenosomes

The fact that the thus far studied protozoal hydrogenosomes and fungal hydrogenosomes seem so different in a number of key aspects may be related to a different origin of the organelle in the two classes of microorganisms.

On the evolutionary origin of hydrogenosomes one can only speculate. Hydrogenosomes from evolutionary ancient protozoa like *T. vaginalis* may be directly derived from bacterial endosymbionts [6,23]. Furthermore it is clear that the presence of hydrogenosomes in diverse phylogenetically unrelated groups indicates the independent acquisition of the organelles on several occasions. How they were acquired, through conversion of already existing (endosymbiont derived) organelles (mitochondria, microbodies?) or whether they represent mainly (all?) primary endosymbiotic events, remains, however, a complete enigma. Finally, hydrogenosomes of anaerobic protozoa and anaerobic fungi are clearly not identical. Many characteristics of protozoal hydrogenosomes are not in accordance with those of microbodies. Nevertheless, to consider them therefore as mitochondria-derived seems also rather premature. The organelles lack as far as we know DNA and even though metabolically they are the anaerobic equivalent of mitochondria, they are equipped with a totally different enzyme complement. Moreover, peroxisomes and probably also other 'true' microbodies do not exclusively use the SKL targeting signal [27]. Thus, by itself the absence of SKL containing proteins in protozoal hydrogenosomes does not form a 100% convincing argument against an evolutionary relationship with peroxisomes, glyoxysomes and glycosomes.

With regard to fungal hydrogenosomes it should be stated that while these organelles do have some characteristics of 'bona fide' microbodies like the presence of proteins which probably contain the typical SKL microbody targeting signal [21], from a metabolic point of view they have, like all hydrogenosomes, nothing in common with other microbodies. Note moreover, that the actual presence and functionality of the SKL targeting signal still need to be established (DNA sequencing data and *in vitro* and/or *in vivo* protein import data should be provided). Finally, Marvin-Sikkema *et al.* [22] observed that the intrahydrogenosomal pH in anaerobic fungi is more basic. Thus in this respect these hydrogenosomes are more analogous to mitochondria than to the peroxisomes which at least in yeast seem somewhat acidic (pH 6,4) [24].

Concluding remarks and perspective

If the pace of development and application of new techniques in this field of research is kept up, we can be sure that the coming years will reveal many exciting new discoveries. Progress in the studies on free-living anaerobic protozoa will benefit from the recent establishment of poly A$^+$ derived cDNA libraries. Specific cDNA's can be isolated and, with cDNA derived primers, subsequently the corresponding genes may be amplified from genomic DNA isolates. In this way the risk of food-bacterial DNA contamination is minimized. PCR amplifying the ferredoxin gene from *P. lanterna* genomic DNA using 5' and 3' oligonucleotide primers derived from the cDNA sequence resulted in products which where indistinguishable from the ferredoxin cDNA (Brul, S & Lauwers, A, unpublished observations). Thus, alike until now studied genes in parasitic flagellates, these first data in a free-living anaerobic amoeboflagellate give no indications for the presence of introns. In *P. lanterna*, genomic restriction enzyme digested DNA was tested in a Southern blot with the homologous ferredoxin gene as probe. Only one band was visualized irrespective of the restriction enzyme used (Brul, S results not shown). Hence, ferredoxin is present in *P. lanterna* as a single copy gene. Similar molecular data for anaerobic fungi are not yet available. In analogy with the studies on e.g. human, rodent and yeast peroxisomes [4,28,29], the availability of mutants lacking functional hydrogenosomes should enable us through complementation analysis after cell fusion to identify key proteins involved in the assembly of a functional hydrogenosome. The generation of anaerobic fungi with an impairment in hydrogenosomal function is currently being pursued. The data which are to be obtained should subsequently enable us to unambiguously place the hydrogenosomes of the various anaerobic eukaryotic microorganisms in the spectrum of known cellular organelles.

Acknowledgements

We would like to thank Prof. Dr. M. Müller for his hospitality during the spring of 1992 which allowed Dr. S. Brul to do initial studies on the molecular biology of *Psalteriomonas lanterna* in his laboratory in New York. Supported by a grant from the Netherlands Organization for Scientific Research (NWO).

References

(1)   Benchimol, M & de Souza W (1983) Fine structure and cytochemistry of the hydrogenosome of *Tritrichomonas foetus*. J. Protozool. 30, 422–425.

(2)   Broers, CAM, Stumm CK & Vogels GD (1989) A heterolobose amoe-boflagellate associated with methanogenic bacteria. In: Lloyd, D, Combs GH & Paget TA (Eds.) Biochemistry and molecular biology of 'anaerobic' protozoa (pp 21–31) Harwood Academic Publishers, London.

(3)   Borst, P (1989) Peroxisome biogenesis revisited. Biochim. Biophys. Acta. 1008, 1–13.

(4)   Brul, S, *et al.* (1988) Genetic heterogeneity in the Cerebro-Hepato-Renal (Zellweger) Syndrome and other inherited disorders with a generalized impairment of peroxisomal functions. A study using com-plementation analysis. J. Clin. Invest. 81, 1710–1715.

(5)   Brul, S., Veltman, RH, Lombardo, MCP & Vogels GD (1994) Molecular cloning of hydrogenosomal ferredoxin cDNA from the anaerobic amoeboflagellate *Psalteriomonas lanterna*. Biochim. Biophys. Acta 1183, 544–546.

(6)   Brul, S & Stumm CK (1994) Symbionts and organelles in anaerobic protozoa and fungi. Trends Ecol. Evol. 9, 319–324.

(7) Goosen, NK, Van Der Drift, C, Stumm, CK & Vogels, GD (1990) End products of metabolism in *Trimyema compressum*. FEMS Microbiol. Lett. 69, 171–176.

(8) SJ, Krisans, S, Keller G-A & Subramani, S (1990) Antibodies directed against the peroxisomal targeting signal of firefly luciferase recognize multiple mammalian peroxisomal proteins. J. Cell Biol. 110, 27–34.

(9) Honigberg, BM, Volkmann, D, Entzeroth, R & Scholtyseck, E (1984) A freeze-fracture electron microscope study of *Trichomonas vaginalis* Donné and *Trichomonas foetus* (Riedmuller). J. Protozool. 31, 116–131.

(10) Johnson, PJ, D'Oliveira, CE, Gorrell, TE & Müller, M (1990) Molecular analysis of the hydrogenosomal ferredoxin of the anaerobic protist *Trichomonas vaginalis* Proc. Natl. Acad. Sci. USA 87, 6097–6101.

(11) Keller, G-A, Krisans, S, Gould, SJ, Sommer, JM, Wang, CC, Schliebs, W, Kunau, W, Brody, S & Subramani, S (1991) Evolutionary conservation of a microbody targeting signal that targets proteins to peroxisomes, glycosomes and glyoxysomes. J. Cell Biol. 114, 893–904.

(12) Lahti, CJ & Johnson, PJ (1991) *Trichomonas vaginalis* hydrogenoso-mal proteins are synthesized on free polyribosomes and may undergo processing upon maturation. Mol. Biochem. Parasitol. 46, 307–310.

(13) Lahti, CJ, D'Oliveira, CE & Johnson, PJ (1992) β-succinyl-coenzyme-A synthetase from *Trichomonas vaginalis* is a soluble hydrogenosomal protein with an amino-terminal sequence that resembles mitochondrial presequences. J. Bacteriol. 174, 6822–6830.

(14) Lahti, CJ, Bradley, PJ & Johnson, PJ (1994) Molecular characterization of the α-subunit of *Trichomonas vaginalis* hydrogenosomal succinyl CoA synthetase. Mol. Biochem. Parasitol. (in press).

(15) Länge, S, Rozario, C & Müller, M (1994) Primary structure of the hydrogenosomal adenylate kinase of *Trichomonas vaginalis* and its phylogenetic relationships. Mol. Biochem. Parasitol. (in press).

(16) Lindmark, DG & Müller, M (1973) Hydrogenosome, a cytoplasmic organelle of the anaerobic flagellate *Tritrichomonas foetus*, and its role in pyruvate metabolism. J. Biol. Chem. 248, 7724–7728.

220 *Hydrogenosomes; Ubiquitous Organelles*

(17) Lindmark, DG, Müller, M & Shio, H (1975) Hydrogenosomes in *Trichomonas vaginalis* J. Parasitol. 63, 552–554.
(18) Lloyd, D, Lindmark DG & Müller, M (1979) Adenosine triphosphatase activity of *Tritrichomonas foetus*. J. Gen. Microbiol. 115, 301–307.
(19) Marczak, R, Gorell, TE & Müller, M (1983) Hydrogenosomal ferredoxin of the anaerobic protozoon *Tritrichomonas foetus*. J. Biol. Chem. 258, 12427–12433.
(20) Marvin-Sikkema, FD, Pedro-Gomez, TM, Grivet, J-P, Gottschal, JC & Prins, RA (1993) Characterization of hydrogenosomes and their role in glucose metabolism of *Neocallimastix* sp. L2. Arch. Microbiol. 160, 388–396.
(21) Marvin-Sikkema, FD, Kraak, MN, Veenhuis, M, Gottschal, JC & Prins, RA (1993) The hydrogenosomal enzyme hydrogenase from the anaerobic fungus *Neocallimastix* sp. L2 is recognized by antibodies directed against the C-terminal microbody protein targeting signal SKL. Eur. J. Cell Biol. 61, 86–91.
(22) Marvin-Sikkema, FD, Driessen, JM, Gottschal, JC & Prins, RA (1994) Metabolic energy generation in hydrogenosomes of the anaerobic fungus *Neocallimastix*: Evidence for a functional relationship with mitochondria. Mycol. Res. (in press).
(23) Müller, M (1993) The Hydrogenosome. J. Gen Microbiol. 139, 2879–2889.
(24) Nicolay, K, Veenhuis, M, Douma, A & Harder, W (1987) A ^{31}P NMR study of the internal pH of yeast peroxisomes. Arch. Microbiol. 147, 37–41.
(25) Nielsen, MH & Diemer, NH (1976) The size, density and relative area of chromatic granules ('hydrogenosomes') in *Trichomonas vaginalis*. Donné from cultures of logarithmic and stationary growth. Cell Tissue Res. 167, 461–465.
(26) Steinbüchel, A & Müller, M (1986) Anaerobic pyruvate metabolism of *Tritrichomonas foetus* and *Trichomonas vaginalis* hydrogenosomes Mol. Biochem. Parasitol. 20, 57–65.
(27) Swinkels, BW, Gould, SJ, Bodnar, RA, Rachubinski, RA & Subramani, S (1991) Identification of a novel peroxisomal targeting signal in the amino-terminal prepiece of 3-ketoacyl-CoA thiolase. J. Cell Biol. 111, 2146–2151.
(28) Tsukamoto, T, Miura, S & Fujiki, Y (1990) Isolation and characterization of Chinese hamster ovary cxell mutants defective in the assembly of peroxisomes. J. Cell Biol. 110, 651–660.
(29) Van Der Lei, I, Van Den Berg, M, Boot, R, Franse, M, Distel B

& Tabak, HF (1992) Isolation of peroxisome assembly mutants from *Saccharomyces cerevisiae* with different morphologies using a novel positive selection procedure. J. Cell Biol. 119, 153–162.

(30) Yarlett, N, Rowlands, C, Yarlett, NC, Evans, JC & Lloyd, D (1987) Respiration of the hydrogenosome containing fungus *Neocallimastix patriciarum*. Arch. Microbiol. 148, 25–28.

(31) Zwart, KB, Goosen, NK, van Schijndel, MW, Broers, CAM, Stumm, CK & Vogels, GD (1988) Cytochemical localization of hydrogenase activity in the anaerobic protozoa *Trichomonas vaginalis*, *Plagiopylanasuta* and *Trimyema compressum*. J. Gen. Microbiol. 134, 2165–2170.

17

BIOGENESIS AND FUNCTION OF HYDROGENOSOMES IN THE ANAEROBIC FUNGUS *NEOCALLIMASTIX* sp. L2; A MOLECULAR APPROACH

W. HARDER and M. VEENHUIS

Biological Center, University of Groningen, Kerklaan 30, 9751 NN Haren, The Netherlands.

Summary

Hydrogenosomes belong to a class of specific subcellular compartments (organelles), called microbodies. The organelles are believed to play an important role in energy metabolism of anaerobic fungi and are involved in the formation of H_2. Recently, evidence has been obtained that the molecular mechanisms involved in sorting and translocation of matrix enzymes probably are conserved between fungal hydrogenosomes and other – e.g. yeast – microbodies. This has opened the way to study hydrogenosome biogenesis and function at the molecular level, taking advantage of the power of yeast genetics. In the past few years numerous yeast mutants have been isolated which are impaired in the biogenesis/function of microbodies (*per* mutants) and several of the corresponding genes have now been cloned and characterized. Cloning of these genes is based on the functional complementation of *per* mutants with a yeast genomic bank. An identical procedure, using *Neocallimastix* cDNAs, will be followed to identify *Neocallimastix PER* genes. In particular we aim to address the fundamental question of the advantage for the fungus to compartmentalize a distinct part of its energy metabolism in hydrogenosomes.

Introduction

Eukaryotic cells contain a number of distinct subcellular compartments (organelles) designed to fulfil specific metabolic functions. Different classes of organelles e.g. nuclei, mitochondria, chloroplasts, vacuoles and endoplasmic reticulum have been (and still are) intensively studied and consequently, much is now known about their biogenesis, specific function in cellular metabolism and mechanisms involved in their functioning. Compared to these, microbodies have drawn relatively little attention. This may be related to the fact that of all ubiquitous cell compartments known, microbodies represent the most recently discovered class, whereas their significance in cellular metabolism was initially considered of minor importance. However, recent studies made the significance of microbodies more clear and showed that, despite their similarity in morphology, the organelles may show a great diversity in enzyme repertoires and, as a consequence, may be involved in a variety of metabolic processes [1–4]. These functions are partly inducible in nature and may vary with the developmental stage and/or growth conditions of the related organism. Their importance in cellular metabolism may be stressed by the fact that in general peroxisomal dysfunctioning leads to severe abnormalities and often is lethal, including in human [5].

Different classes of microbodies, summarized in Table 17.1, have now been identified. At present, the knowledge of hydrogenosome biogenesis/function is hardly beyond the descriptive level. However, recently evidence has been obtained that sorting of hydrogenosomal matrix proteins may proceed by mechanisms which are similar to those described for peroxisomes and glycosomes [8]. This indicates that the molecular machinery involved in microbody biogenesis may at least in part be conserved between hydrogenosomes and throughout other members of the microbody family. This has now opened the way to study various aspects of hydrogenosome biogenesis and function at the molecular level, taking advantage of the power of yeast genetics.

In this contribution we will summarize different recent achievements on yeast microbodies which are relevant to this topic and present the strategy, which will be followed by identifying *Neocallimastix* genes which are essential for hydrogenosome biogenesis/function.

Table 17.1   DIFFERENT TYPES OF MICROBODIES IN EUKARYOTES

Organelle	Organism	Key enzymes	Reference
hydrogenosome	ciliates, anaerobic fungi	hydrogenase	6
peroxisome	animals, plants, fungi	catalase, oxidases	2
glyoxysome	plants, yeast	glyoxylate cycle	3
glycosome	Kinetoplastida	glycolytic enzymes	7

Yeast microbodies (peroxisomes, glyoxysomes)

GENERAL PROPERTIES OF MICROBODIES

1. Induction and metabolic function of microbodies. Microbodies are distinguished from other cell organelles by their relatively simple morphology. In general they are irregular or rounded in shape, measure up to 1.5 µm, contain a homogeneous protein-aceous matrix which may contain crystalline inclusions and are surrounded by a single membrane [1]. In yeasts the proliferation and metabolic significance of microbodies (peroxisomes, glyoxysomes) is largely prescribed by environmental stimuli (e.g. growth conditions). Well known examples of microbody proliferation are those described for cells grown in the presence of fatty acids, methanol, C_{2-} compounds like ethanol, primary amines, D-amino acids or purines [2]. In the yeast *Hansenula polymorpha* optimal induction is achieved during methylotrophic growth conditions (when microbodies may constitute up to 80% of the cytoplasmic volume).

    A characteristic feature of the organelles is that they contain key enzymes of the metabolism of the above compounds (for reviews see 1–4). Based on our current knowledge of microbody proliferation in yeasts we are now able to precisely adjust both the level of microbody induction as well as their protein composition by selecting appropriate growth conditions.

2. Development of microbodies. It is now generally accepted that upon their induction by certain growth substrates, microbodies (peroxisomes) in yeast develop from pre-existing organelles by fission. Precursors of matrix proteins, encoded by nuclear genes, are synthesized on free polysomes in the cytosol and are post-translationally imported without further processing and assembled into active enzymes in the peroxisomal matrix. Topogenic signals, directing peroxisomal matrix proteins to their target organelle reside in the mature protein sequence. The first microbody targeting signal (PTS) was identified in 1989 in firefly luciferase and appeared to consist of three amino acids (SKL), located at the extreme carboxy terminus of the protein [9]. Subsequent studies indicated that the SKL (or SKL-like)-motive is also effective as PTS in a wide range of other organisms, suggesting that the cellular machinery to recognize this or comparable tripeptide C-terminal sequences may be highly conserved in eukaryotic cells [10].

However, it is certainly not the only sequence acting as such because many of the known microbody matrix enzymes lack this motive. Moreover, in a few matrix enzymes (e.g. thiolase and amine oxidase) the targeting information is shown to reside in the extreme N-terminus of the protein. The targeting signals for the major peroxisomal matrix proteins of methanol-grown *H. polymorpha*, namely alcohol oxidase (AO) and dihydroxyacetone synthase (DHAS) have also been identified. Both signals are again tripeptides, located at the extreme C-terminus of the proteins and comprise the sequence N-K-L-COOH for DHAS and A-R-F-COOH for AO [11,12]. Very recently, Marvin-Sikkema et al. [8] demonstrated that the hydrogenase in *Neocallimastix* contained a C-terminal SKL-motive. This important finding indicates that the mechanisms involved in sorting and translocation of microbody matrix proteins are conserved between yeasts and anaerobic fungi.

BIOGENESIS OF PEROXISOMES

1. Mutant isolation and characterization. A series of mutants of *H. polymorpha* affected in the biogenesis/assembly of peroxisomes have been isolated and characterized [11]. Phenotypically these mutants are characterized by the fact that they are not able to grow on methanol (Mut⁻-phenotype). Within the collection of Mut⁻ mutants obtained, three main classes of peroxisomal mutant phenotypes were identified i) *peroxisomal im*port mutants, morphologically characterized by the presence of few small peroxisomes in conjunction with a major fraction of peroxisomal matrix enzymes in the cytosol (Pim⁻ mutants; 5 complementation groups), ii) *per*oxisome deficient mutants which completely lack recognizable peroxisomal structures (Per⁻-mutants, 13 complementation groups) and iii) mutants which displayed gross aberrations in *per*oxisomal *sub*structure, most probably due to improper assembly of part of the matrix protein (Pss⁻ phenotype; 7 strains). In addition several conditional Per⁻, Pim⁻ and Pss⁻ mutants (temperature sensitive [ts], cold sensitive [cs] and pH-sensitive mutants) have been isolated.

    Backcrossing experiments revealed that all *per* mutant phenotypes are due to monogenetic defects, which implies that the absence (or incorrect synthesis) of a single gene product may cause the absence of a complete organelle (the peroxisome). This unique property renders these mutants very attractive for a molecular analysis of peroxisome biogenesis. The latter was convincingly illustrated by our studies on *perts* mutants [12]. These mutants are not able to grow on methanol and show the Per⁻ phenotype at the restrictive temperature (43°C) but have wild type properties (and contain normal peroxisomes) at permissive growth conditions (<37°C). Interestingly, at intermediate temperatures (between 37–43°C) the cells displayed the Pim⁻ phenotype, the number and size of peroxisomes being directly related to the temperature and thus, to the level of expression of the ts- gene; therefore, these may be considered an intermediary defect in peroxisome biogenesis.

Physiologically, *per* mutants are characterized by the fact that they are not able to grow on methanol (Mut⁻) as the sole carbon source. However, in the *per* mutants analyzed so far, the various peroxisomal matrix and membrane proteins are normally synthesized and assembled into the active protein in the cytosol of these cells [11,13]. Thus, also alcohol oxidase is normally present and organized in a large cytosolic crystalloid (Fig. 17.1) together with other matrix enzymes like dihydroxyacetone synthase [14]. Detailed biochemical and physiological studies of these cells revealed that nevertheless the presence of intact peroxisomes is a prerequisite to enable growth of the organism on methanol. The results obtained revealed that the indispensable functions of intact peroxisomes in methanol metabolism are twofold namely i) to control the proper partitioning of formaldehyde fluxes (generated from methanol) over dissimilatory and assimilatory pathways and ii) to facilitate decomposition (by catalase) of hydrogen peroxide at the site where it is produced thus preventing hydrogen peroxide decomposition by other – energy consuming – processes [15]. In contrast, growth on glucose in the presence of various organic nitrogen sources (e.g. primary amines or D-amino acids) which require the activity of peroxisome-borne enzymes in WT cells, is fully unaffected [16]. Thus, certain peroxisomal pathways can effectively function in the cytosol in these mutants. *H. polymorpha* mutants displaying a Per⁻ phenotype also were able to grow on ethanol. However, both the growth rate and final yield is reduced compared to wild type controls. Detailed physiological studies suggested that the main advantage of intact microbodies in ethanol-metabolism is that it enables the cell to adjust the levels of different intermediates required to generate aspartate (the final product of microbody C_2-metabolism) from isocitrate. In particu-

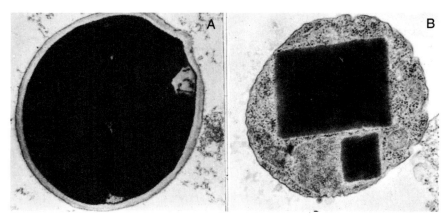

Figure 17.1. Survey of cells of *Hansenula polymorpha* showing the overall cell morphology of WT (a) and peroxisome-deficient (b) cells after growth in continuous cultures (D = 0.07h^{-1}) on glucose/ methanol mixtures. In the WT cell approximately 20 peroxisomal profiles are visualized. In the per mutant a large cytosolic crystalloid is present, composed of alcohol oxidase protein. A smaller crystalloid is located in the nucleus. The cells are fixed with KMnO$_4$ (a) or glutaraldehyde/OsO$_4$ (b).

lar, the intact organelles may prevent a drain of oxaloacetate into other metabolic pathways. Summarizing, these results indicate that the advantage of the presence of functional peroxisomes varies with the compounds used for growth. The general reason as to why different metabolic pathways are located in microbodies may therefore mainly be the advantage of compartmentalizing the formation of a certain metabolic intermediate with the enzyme for which this should subsequently serve as a substrate, thereby preventing a drain of the intermediate to other metabolic pathways.

2.   Cloning of genes essential for peroxisome biogenesis. Extensive complementation analysis of mutant strains bearing single recessive mutations in either of twelve yet identified *PER* genes (*PER1-PER12*) revealed many cases of 'non-complementation': diploids containing both WT and mutant alleles of two different *PER* genes displayed mutant phenotypes which were predominantly observed at lowered temperatures (cold-sensitive non-complementation). The combined data on unlinked non-complementation events enabled us to construct a map [17] of genetic interactions between the twelve *PER* genes (Fig. 17.2).

For cloning of the different *PER* genes by functional complementation of per mutants of *H. polymorpha* efficient transformation systems have been developed, offering transformation frequencies of 10^5 to 10^6

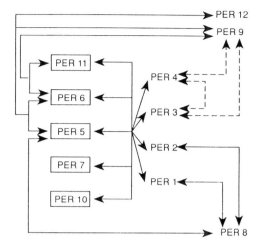

Figure 17.2. Interactions between products of *PER1* to *PER12* genes deduced from unlinked non-complementation data. The dotted lines indicate 'weak' interactions ('leaky' growth of the corresponding double heterozygous hybrids at restrictive temperatures).

transformants per μg plasmid DNA. By means of functional complementation of selected *per* mutants (using a *H. polymorpha* genomic bank and restoration to the Mut+ phenotype as selection criterion) seven *PER* genes have now been cloned and are currently characterized. One of the cloned genes was found to encode for a protein involved in microbody protein recognition/translocation and appeared to represent the *H. polymorpha* homologue of PAS8 from *Pichia pastoris*, the gene product of which is suggested to act as the SKL receptor [18]. Since, as indicated above, SKL or SKL-like signals also may function in fungal hydrogenosomes [8], different protein components which play a role in hydrogenosome matrix protein recognition/translocation may have functional equivalents in yeast.

Therefore, the different ingredients required to initiate molecular studies on hydrogenosome biogenesis/function in a fashion similar to the above strategy followed for yeasts, are now available.

Our prime objective is to develop the tools to manipulate the proper assembly of hydrogenosomes in the anaerobic fungus *Neocallimastix* sp L2 with the aim

i) to identify and characterize protein components essential for the biogenesis of hydrogenosomes and

ii) to elucidate the significance of intact hydrogenosomes in the intermediary metabolism of the fungus with emphasis on the specific advantage for the organism to compartmentalize metabolic pathways in this organelle.

Biogenesis and function of hydrogenosomes in *Neocallimastix* sp L2; a structure/function analysis

MORPHOLOGICAL STUDIES

The ultrastructure of hydrogenosmes in intact hyphae and zoospores of *Neocallimastix* will be analyzed in depth using different advanced methods e.g. freeze substitution. This way information will be obtained on i) the proliferation of the organelles in relation to environmental conditions and ii) eventual structural adaptations of the organelle in, for instance, shape and formation of additional internal membranes related to organellar functioning.

IDENTIFICATION OF *NEOCALLIMASTIX* HOMOLOGUES OF *H. POLYMORPHA* PER GENES

The strategy for the cloning of genes essential for hydrogenosome biogenesis is based on the functional complementation of selected peroxisome-deficient (*per*) mutants of *H. polymorpha* using *Neocallimastix* genomic or cDNAs cloned in a suitable *H. polymorpha* expression vector [19].

   We will elucidate the function(s) of the encoded proteins by sequencing the genes and perform sequence comparisons with the yeast homologues cloned so far (*Pichia pastoris, S.cerevisae* and *H.polymorpha*) and DNA and protein databases (search for functional domains), and by characterizing the encoded proteins (e.g. location in the cell, regulation of expression). Functional tests will also be performed in constructed conditional mutants of the yeast, in which the gene of interest is placed under control of a substrate-inducible promotor. For this purpose both the alcohol oxidase and the amine oxidase promotor are available.

CONSTRUCTION OF *NEOCALLIMASTIX* MUTANTS IMPAIRED IN HYDROGENOSOME FUNCTION/ASSEMBLY

Two types of *Neocallimastix* mutants will be constructed namely i) by disruption of the *Neocallimastix PER* genes, obtained as described above in section b and ii) by deleting the targeting signal (SKL) of the matrix key enzyme hydrogenase.

Both types of mutants will be analyzed in detail with respect to growth and physiological/biochemical properties and will provide insight in the specific role of the intact hydrogenosome in different metabolic functions.

References

(1) BORST, P. (1989). Peroxisome biogenesis revisited. Biochim. Biophys. Acta, 1008:1–13.

(2) FAHIMI, H.D. and SIES, H. (1987). Peroxisomes in Biology and Medicine. Springer-Verlag Berlin Heidelberg.

(3) VEENHUIS, M. and HARDER, W. (1988). Microbodies in yeasts: structure, function and biogenesis. Microbiol. Sci. 5: 347–351.

(4) VEENHUIS, M. and HARDER, W. (1991). Microbodies. p. 601–653. *In* A. Rose (ed.), The Yeasts, vol. 4. Acad. Press.

(5) WANDERS, R.J.A., HEYMANS, H.S.A., SCHUTGENS, R.B.H., BARTH, P.G., VAN DEN BOSCH, H. and TAGER, J.M. (1988). Peroxisomal disorders in neurology. J. Neurol. Sci. 88:1–39.

(6) LINDMARK, D.G. and MÜLLER, M. (1973). Hydrogenosome, a cytoplasmic organelle of the anaerobic flagellate *Tritrichomonas foetus*, and its role in pyruvate metabolism. J. Biol. Chem. 248 :7724–7728

(7) OPPERDOES, F.R. and BORST, P. (1977). Localization of nine glycolytic enzymes in a microbody-like organelle in *Trypanosoma brucei*: the glycosome. FEBS Letters 80: 360–364

(8) MARVIN-SIKKEMA, F.D., KRAAK, M.N., VEENHUIS, M., GOTTSCHAL, J.C. and PRINS, R.A. (1993). The hydrogenosomal enzyme hydrogenase from the anaerobic fungus *Neocallimastix* sp.L2 is recognized by antibodies directed against the C-terminal microbody protein targeting signal SKL. Eur. J. Cell Biol. 61: 86–91.

(9) GOULD, S.J., KELLER, G.A. and SUBRAMANI, S. (1988). Identification of peroxisomal targeting signals at the carboxy terminus of four peroxisomal proteins. J. Cell Biol. 107: 897–905.

(10) SUBRAMANI, S. (1992). Targeting of proteins into the peroxisomal matrix. J. Membr. Biol. 125: 99–106.

(11)   VEENHUIS, M. (1992). Peroxisome biogenesis and function in*Hansenula polymorpha*. Cell Biochem. Funct. 10: 175–184.

(12)   WATERHAM, H.W., SWAVING, G.J., TITORENKO, V., HARDER, W. and VEENHUIS, M. (1993). Peroxisomes in the methylotrohpic yeast *Hansenula polymorpha* do not necessarily derive from pre-existing organelles. EMBO J. 12: 4785 – 4794.

(13)   SULTER, G.J., VRIELING, E.G., HARDER, W. and VEEN-HUIS, M. (1993). Synthesis and subcellular location of peroxisomal membrane proteins in a peroxisome-deficient mutant of the yeast *Hansenula polymorpha*. EMBO J. 12: 2205–2210.

(14)   VAN DER KLEI, I.J., SULTER, G.J., HARDER, W. and VEENHUIS, M. (1991). Expression, assembly and crystallization of alcohol oxidase in a peroxisome-deficient mutant of *Hansenula polymorpha*; properties of the protein and architecture of the crystals. Yeast 7: 15–24.

(15)   VAN DER KLEI, I.J., HARDER, W. and VEENHUIS, M. (1991). Methanol metabolism in a peroxisome-deficient mutant of *Hansenula polymorpha*: a physiological study. Arch. Microbiol. 156: 15–23.

(16)   SULTER, G.J., VAN DER KLEI, I.J., HARDER, W. and VEENHUIS, M. (1990). Expression and assembly of amine oxidase and D-amino acid oxidase in the cytoplasm of peroxisome-deficient mutants of the yeast *Hansenula polymorpha* during growth on primary amines or D-alanine as the sole nitrogen source. YEAST 6: 501–507.

(17)   TITORENKO, V., WATERHAM, H.R., CREGG, J.M., HARDER, W. and VEENHUIS, M (1993). A complex set of interacting genes controls peroxisome biogenesis in *Hansenula polymorpha*. PNAS USA 90: 7470–7474.

(18)   MCCOLLUM, D., MONOSOV, E. and SUBRAMAINI, S. (1993). The *pas*8 mutant of *Pichia pastoris* exhibits the peroxisomal protein import deficiencies of Zellweger Syndrome cells – The PAS8 protein binds to the COOH-terminal tripeptide peroxisomal targeting signal, and is a member of the TPR protein family. J. Cell Biol. 121: 761–774.

(19)   FABER, K.N., SWAVING, G.J., FABER, F., AB, G., HARDER, W., VEENHUIS, M. and HAIMA, P. (1992). Chromosomal targeting of replicating plasmids in the yeast *Hansenula polymorpha*. J. Gen. Microbiol. 138: 2405–2416.

OVERVIEW AND RECOMMENDATIONS

Much progress was made in the past by treating the rumen as a black box, and learning about its contribution to the animal more or less empirically. It is our view that in the long term, understanding how the rumen microbes degrade plant cell walls to produce microbial protein, volatile fatty acids, CO_2 and methane should allow us to control these and other processes that occur in the rumen to the benefit of agrarian and agro-industrial communities world-wide. Here, the distribution and nature of plant resources have been considered, together with the functions of the rumen microorganisms, with special (but not exclusive) reference to the possible roles of the anaerobic fungi in plant cell wall hydrolysis and in methanogenesis via the production of hydrogen.

Plant resources

Consideration of the resources available for ruminant feeds identified the problem of transporting bulky forages from the major growing areas to centres of animal production. In addition, the presence in some forages of toxic secondary metabolites is a major constraint to their utilization. The successful protection of Australian ruminants from *Leucaena* toxicity by the introduction of toxin degrading bacteria from Hawaii and from Indonesia offers hope that further characterization of the toxic metabolites of plants and studies on microbial transformation of plant secondary metabolites will lead to the development of strategies for detoxification in the rumen, releasing new resources for use as ruminant feeds.

Rumen fungi-interrelationships with other rumen microorganisms

It has been shown that rumen fungi interact with other components of the rumen flora in different ways. Some bacteria, particularly those that act as hydrogen sinks such as the methanogens, appear to stimulate fermentation and growth by the fungi, and thus increase their cellulolytic activity. Other bacteria produce factors inhibitory to the fungi, reducing their ability to ferment cellulose. These interactions

233

suggest that the activity of the fungi in the rumen might be susceptible to manipulation once the true nature of the various interactions are understood. For example, the supply of alternative hydrogen sinks might reduce the activity of the methanogens, but maintain high fermentative activity of the fungi. The inhibitors from *Ruminococcus flavefaciens* (or more probably chemicals synthesized to exert the same effects) could be used to study the effect of removal of the fungi on the dynamics and productivity of the rumen fermentation. The use of gnotobiotic ruminants offers the opportunity for further studies on the interactions between the anaerobic fungi and other rumen microorganisms.

Applications of molecular biology

A wide range of molecular biological techniques is being used to increase our understanding about how the rumen fungi function. The first priority is the development of transformation systems for anaerobic fungi; this is likely to be difficult as there are relatively few such systems available for aerobic fungi despite many years of research effort. However, current knowledge of the genetics of the yeast *Hansenula* provides a way forward, by complementation experiments. Experiments are in progress to introduce cDNA (DNA formed from RNA) from the anaerobic fungi into *Hansenula* mutants to isolate certain fungal genes.

The separation and purification of enzymes, including both those involved in intermediary metabolism and the extracellular cellulases and xylanases, has proved difficult, and is already being aided by molecular cloning, by which means single gene products can be expressed in bacteria like *Escherichia coli* that are easy to grow. Molecular methods will also allow us to study the regulation of gene expression in the fungi, by determining at which stages in the life cycle or under which environmental conditions particular genes are transcribed.

Molecular studies in rumen bacteria such as *Prevotella* and *Ruminococcus flavefaciens* are well advanced, but there is no significant knowledge of the molecular biology of the rumen protozoa or the rumen fungi.

Hydrogenases and hydrogenosomes

Consideration of the biology and origins of hydrogenosomes suggest that the study of hydrogen production by bacteria, and particularly by

Clostridium, may have important clues for us in our attempts to understand how the fungi produce hydrogen. Similarities in leader peptides (SKL sequences) between hydrogenosomal proteins of anaerobic fungi and peroxisomal proteins of aerobic fungi have hinted at a possible evolutionary relationships between these organellles; in contrast, the hydrogenosomes of anaerobic protozoa appear different from those of the fungi. The demonstration of ATPases in hydrogenosomes suggests that these organelles have a very important role in the energy metabolism of the fungi. The mechanisms involved in transport across the hydrogenosomal membranes need to be elucidated (here again the similarities with bacteria may hold important clues) and the consequences for the fungi of the loss of their hydrogenases by mutations could reveal more about the role of these enzymes in fungal metabolism.

Plant cell wall degradation

The production by anaerobic rumen fungi of some of the most active cellulases known to man is an obvious reason for studying these microorganisms and their enzymes in detail. Molecular studies have proved particularly valuable and despite the low GC ratio of fungal DNA and the presence of introns (non-coding regions) in some sequences, genes coding for key enzymes have been cloned and expressed in bacteria for detailed study. These enzymes are of considerable commercial interest in a variety of industrial applications, but they may also prove to be useful in ruminant nutrition. Recent work in the USA has suggested that the addition to the ruminant diet of certain enzymes, especially phenolic acid esterases but by implication other enzymes too, may increase the rate of fermentation of fibre in the rumen. It can be argued that because the rumen bacteria degrade plant fibre by means of membrane associated systems like cellulosomes, there is a digestion lag on first introduction of fibre into the rumen prior to bacterial colonization and proliferation. The addition of enzymes complementary to those of the rumen microflora is thought to shorten this lag and increase the rate of fermentation. Anaerobic fungi possess highly active phenolic acid esterases and the industrial production of fungal enzymes for addition to ruminant diets may prove to be both feasible and profitable. Other comparable enzymes, such as those from the anaerobic bacterium *Ruminococcus flavefaciens*, may also have similar application.

Future research priorities

Evolution has been accompanied by biological diversification and the division of labour between different organisms or the formation of cell compartments within single organisms. It is interesting that when we consider the possible genetic manipulation of microorganisms to enhance processes in the rumen and other natural system, we often propose to put evolution into reverse, and produce strains able to carry out reactions that in nature would be achieved by a mixed population. Presumably, evolution has tried and generally failed with this strategy (otherwise the diversity of microbial forms that we can see today would be relatively limited) and we should learn from that! Genetic manipulation has proved to be an excellent means of investigating microbial function and for the production of industrial products under controlled conditions, but society will probably impose limitations on the release of manipulated 'superbugs' into the environment: in the meantime there are several obvious major areas for further work highlighted by the present meeting. These include a number of priorities.

- Identification of plant toxic factors and use of microbial transformation in the rumen.
- Study and application of fungal enzymes, especially those involved in plant cell wall degradation.
- Application of the *Hansenula* complementation system (or other yeast/fungal systems) to study gene function in the fungi.
- Development of transformation systems for further studies on fungal genetics.
- Elucidation of the life cycle of the fungi to demonstrate the nature of resistant structures that ensure the survival of these organisms in nature. This would facilitate maintenance and distribution of stock cultures, necessary if the fungi are to be used industrially.
- Production of hydrogenase-less mutants as part of investigation of the role of hydrogen production in the growth of fungi
- Identification of microbial or non-microbial electron sinks to compete with methanogens.
- Characterization of cell wall components of anaerobic fungi, especially in relation to phylogeny, the role of surface receptors in substrate utilization and adhesion to surfaces.

LIST OF PARTICIPANTS

DENMARK

Dr. M.R. Weisbjerg
National Institute of Animal Sciences
Department of Research in Cattle and Sheep
Foulum, Postbus 39
8830 Tjele
Denmark

Fax No. 89 99 13 00
Tel: 89 99 19 00

FRANCE

Dr. A. Breton
Institut Universitaire de Technologie
Département 'Analyses Biologiques et Biochimiques'
Ensemble Univeristaire des Cézeaux
PO 86
63 172 Aubiere Cedex
France

Fax No. 73 40 76 70
Tel: 73 40 74 74

Dr. R. Durand
Centre de Génétique Moléculaire et Cellulaire
Université Lyon 1
Bât 405 – 43
Boulevard du 11 Novembre 1918
69622 Villeurbanne Cedex
France

Fax No. 72 43 11 81
Tel: 72 43 83 78

Dr. M. Fevre
Centre de Génétique Moléculaire et Cellulaire
Université Lyon 1

Bât 405 – 43
Boulevard du 11 Novembre 1918
69622 Villeurbanne Cedex
France

Fax No. 72 43 11 81
Tel: 72 44 83 78

Dr. G. Fonty
Institut National de la Recherche Agronomique
Laobratoire de Microbiologie
Centre de Recherches de Clermont-Ferrand
Theix 63122
St Genes Champanelle
France

Fax No. 73 62 44 50
Tel: 73 62 40 00

Dr. Ph. Gouet
Institut National de la Recherche Agronomique
Laobratoire de Microbiologie
Centre de Recherches de Clermont-Ferrand
Theix 63122
St Genes Champanelle
France

Fax No. 73 62 44 50
Tel: 73 62 40 00

Dr. J-P. Jouany
Station de Recherches sur la Nutrition des Herbivores
Unite Digestion Microbienne
INRA Centre de Recherches de Clermont-Ferrand/Theix
63122 Saint Genes Champanelle
France

Fax No. 73 62 44 50
Tel: 73 62 40 00

GERMANY

Dr. J. Brinkmann
Institute fur Tierphysiologie und Tierernhrung

Kellnerweg 6
G-337077 Gottingen
Germany

Fax No. 55 13 93 408
Tel: 55 13 93 343

GREECE

Dr. G. Zervas
Agricultural University of Athens
Department of Animal Nutrition
IERA ODOS 75
Athens 11855
Greece

Fax No. 13 47 14 76
Tel: 13 47 09 57

IRELAND

Dr. P. O'Keily
Teagasc
Grange Research Centre
Dunsany
Co. Meath
Eire

Fax No. 4 62 51 87
Tel: 4 62 52 14

ITALY

Dr. F. Martillotti
Instituo Sperimentale per la Zootecnia
Bezione Foraggi E Mangimi
Via Salaria 31
Rome
Italy

Fax No. 6 90 615 41
Tel: 6 90 615 47

Professor G. Moniello
Universita Degli Studi di Napoli Federico II
Dipartimento di Scienze Zootechniche
80137 Napoli
Via Delpino 1
Italy

Fax No. 81 29 29 81
Tel: 432 65 01 10

Professor P. Susmel
Departimento di Scienze Della Produzione Animale
Universita Degli Studi di Udine
Facolta di Agraria
33010 Pagnacco 11
Villa Rizzani – via S. Mauro 2
Italy

Fax No. 43 26 60 614
Tel: 43 26 50 110

PORTUGAL

Professor J. Abreu
Instituto Superior de Agronomia
Departmento de Producao Agricola e Animal
Universidade Technica de Lisboa
1399 Lisboa Cedex
Portugal

Fax No. 13 36 35 031
Tel: 13 36 38 161

SPAIN

Dr. J.A. Leal
Centro de Investigaciones Biologicas
Velazquez 144
28006 Madrid
Spain

Fax No. 1 562 75 18
Tel: 1 561 18 00

THE NETHERLANDS

Dr. S. Brul
Unilever Research Laboratory,
Research and Engineering Division
Section Microbiology and Hygienic Processing
Olivier van Noortlaan 120 NL 3133
AT Vlaardingen
The Netherlands

Fax No. 10 460 5800
Tel: 10 460 5173

Dr. H. Op den Camp
Department of Microbiologie
University of Nijmegen
Toernooiveld 6525 ED
Nijmegen
The Netherlands

Fax No. 80 55 34 50
Tel: 80 65 32 15

Dr. R. Dijkerman
Department of Microbiologie
University of Nijmegen
Toernooiveld 6525 ED
Nijmegen
The Netherlands

Fax No. 80 55 34 50
Tel: 80 65 32 15

Dr. M. van der Giezen
Rijksuniversiteit Groningen
Biologisch Centrum
Laboratorium voor Microbiologie
Kerklaan 30
9751 NN Haren
The Netherlands

Fax No. 50 63 21 54
Tel: 50 63 21 50

Dr. J.C. Gottschal
Department of Microbiology
Biology Centre-Haren
University of Groningen
PO Box 14
9750 Haren
The Netherlands

Fax No. 50 63 21 54
Tel: 50 63 21 62

Dr. W. Harder
Rijskuniversiteit Groningen
Afd. Elektronenmiroscopie
Biologisch Centrum
Kerklaan 30
9751 NN Haren
The Netherlands

Fax No. 50 63 52 05
Tel: 50 63 21 50

Dr. H. Marvin
Centrum voor Plantenveredelings-en
Reproduktieonderzoek (CPRO-DLO)
Centrum voor Genetishce
Bronnen Nederland
Droevendaalsesteeg 1
Postbus 6
6700 AA Wageningen
The Netherlands

Fax No. 83 70 1 80 94
Tel: 83 70 70 00

Professor R.A. Prins
Department of Microbiology
Biology Centre-Haren
University of Groningen
PO Box 14
9750 Haren
The Netherlands

Fax No. 50 63 21 54
Tel: 50 53 21 50

Dr. M. Veenhuis
Rijskuniversiteit Groningen
Afd. Elektronenmicroscopie
Biologisch Centrum
Kerklaan 30
9751 NN Haren
The Netherlands
Fax No. 50 63 52 05
Tel: 50 63 21 50

Dr. G.D. Vogels
Department of Microbiology
Faculty of Science
University of Nijmegen
Toernooiveld
NL-6525 ED
Nijmegen
The Netherlands
Fax No. 80 55 34 50
Tel: 80 65 29 41

Dr. F. Voncken
Department of Microbiologie
University of Nijmegen
Toernooiveld 6525 ED
Nijmegen
The Netherlands
Fax No. 80 55 34 50
Tel: 80 65 32 15

UNITED KINGDOM

Dr. H.J. Flint
Rowett Research Institute Greenburn Road
Bucksburn
Aberdeen
United Kingdom
Fax No. 224 716687
Tel: 224 716651

Dr. C.S. Stewart
Rowett Research Institute Greenburn Road
Bucksburn
Aberdeen
United Kingdom

Fax No. 224 716687
Tel: 224 716654

Dr. A.P.J. Trinci
Cryptogamic Botany Laboratories
Department of Botany
University of Manchester
Manchester M13 9PL
United Kingdom

Fax No. 61 275 5656
Tel: 61 275 3893

INDEX

Acetaldehyde dehydrogenase 180, 187–188, 211
Acetate 102, 180–191, 195, 197, 210–212
Acetate:succinate CoA transferase 180, 184, 186, 197, 211
Acetylene 186
Acetyl xylan xesterase 50, 54
Adaptation, bacterial 22
Adenylate kinase 180, 186, 188, 212–213
 -inhibition 188
ADP/ATPtranslocase 179–180, 184, 189–190
 -inhibition 189–190
Aggregation, microbial 22
Alanine aminotransferase 15
Alcohol dehydrogenase 180, 187–188, 211
Alcohol oxidase, targeting signal 226
Aldolase 211
Ammonia
 -emissions 30–31
 -rumen 44–47, 70, 75–76
Amylase 113, 114
Anaeromyces elegans 83
A. mucronatus 83, 99, 172
α-L-Arabinofuranosidase 50, 106
Aradopsis 143
Aspergillus clavatus 158
A. flavipes 158
A. fumigatus 158
A. nidulans 86, 158
A. niger 158
A. ochraceus 158
A. ornatus 158
Aspergillus cell walls 153–162
ATPase 179–180, 188–190
 -inhibition 179, 188–190
Avicelase 56, 117–120

Barley 2, 4
Biogenesis
 -hydrogenosome 215–216, 230–231
 -peroxisome 226–229

Blastocladiella emersonii 140
Brassica napus 19
Buffer capacity, rumen 43–47
Butyrivibrio fibrisolvens 21, 52–60

Caecomyces communis 83, 86, 98–100, 172, 183
C. equi 83, 85–86, 172
Caldocellum saccharolyticum 57
Candida albicans 138, 142–143, 146, 201
Carbon monoxide 187–188
Carboxymethylcellulase 15, 106, 115–122
Catabolite regulation 115
Cellobiohydrolase
 -see exoglucanase
β-D-Cellobiosidase 106
Cellodextrinase 53, 56
Cellulase 106
 -see avicelase, cellulosome,
  carboxymethylcellulase,
  cellodextrinase, exo-glucanase,
  endo-glucanase, glucohydrolase
Cellulose 51, 115
 -amount in forage CW 9
 -degradation 69–77
Cellulosome 54, 55, 121
Clitocybe geotrapa lectin (CGL) 169
Clostridium thermocellum 54–56, 192
Clover 2, 4
Comptonia peregrina 15
Concanavalin A 20
p-Coumaric acid 15, 29–42
 -extraction procedure 38
Coumarin (1, 2 benzopyrone) 15
Crop
 -production 1–10
 -animal feeds 5–6

Dasytricha 19, 103
Datura stramonium lectin (DSL) 169, 172–174
Diethylstilbestrol 179, 189–190

245

Dihydroxyacetone synthase, targeting
   signal 226
Diospyros virginiana 15
Drosophila 143

Embden-Meyerhof-Parnas pathway 179–
   192, 196–197, 210–212
Endo-glucanase 50, 53–57, 59, 113, 114–
   122, 129
Enolase 137–149, 180, 184, 211
   -gene 138–149
   -sequence, nucleotide 139–142
   -sequence, amino acid 142–143
Endocytosis 201–203
Entodinium 19, 69–75
Epidinium 69–75
Escherichia coli 214
Ethanol 99, 179–185, 190, 197, 211–212
Eubacterium limosum 102
Eudiplodinium 69–73
Eupenicillium angustiporcatum 158
E. baarnense 158
E. catenatum 158
E. cinnamopurpureum 158
E. crustaceum 154, 158
E. cryptum 158
E. inusitatum 158
E. lapidosum 158
E. ochro-salmoneum 158
E. parvum 158
E. pinetorum 158
E. shearii 158
E. sinaicum 158
E. stolkiae 158
E. terrenum 158
Eupenicillium cell walls 153–162
Evolution
   -eukaryotes 196–199
   -hydrogenosomes 199–203, 216–218
Exo-glucanase 50, 53–57, 113, 114–122

Feed utilization 5–6
Fermentation
   -products, fungal 99, 117, 180–185,
      190–191, 211–212
   -pathways, see Embden-Meyerhof-
      Parnas pathway
Ferulic acid 15, 29–42
   -extraction procedure 38

Fibrobacter succinogenes 21, 51–60, 99, 106
Formate 99, 179–184, 191, 197, 211–121
β-Fucosidase 113, 114, 129
Fumarase 180, 211
Fumarate reductase 180, 187–188, 211
Fungi, anaerobic
   -antibodies to 87
   -classification 81–83
   -distribution 79–81
   -life cycle 84–89
   -numbers 44, 46
   -gas production 88–89
   -see *Neocallimastix, Piromyces, Piromonas,
      Caecomyces, Sphaeromonas, Orpinomyces,
      Anaeromyces*

Galactofuranans, fungal 153–162
   -extraction & isolation 155–156
   -analysis 157
   -structure & distribution 157–162
β-Galactosidase 129
Gliocladium viride 154
Glucohydrolase 113–115
α-D-Glucosidase 106
β-D-Glucosidase 15, 50, 106, 113, 114–
   121, 129
α-Glucuronidase 50
Glutamate ammonia ligase 15
Glycerol 3-phosphate dehydrogenase 211
Glycerol 3-phosphatase 211
Glycosome 224
Glyoxisome 224–226
Gnotobiotic sheep 105–107
Grasses 2, 4
   -chemical composition 8
   -intake 8
Grassland 2, 4
   -chemical composition 8
   -intake 8

Hansenula polymorpha 225–230
Hemicellulose 17, 51, 128
   -acetylation 17
   -amount in forage CW 9
Hemicellulase 106, 114–122
   -see xylanase
Hexokinase 180, 184, 187, 211
Hydrocinnamic acids 17
Hydrogen 20, 102, 107, 179–183, 187,

190–191, 195, 197, 209–211, 215, 223

Hydrogenase, fungal 179–192, 197, 211
-inhibitors 187–188

Hydrogenosome
-fungal 179–192, 195–203, 209–218
-protozoal 209–218

p-Hydroxybenzoic acid 29, 36–37

p-Hydroxyphenylacetic acid 29, 35–37

3–4 Hydroxyphenylpropionic acid 29, 35–37

Induction, enzyme 55, 130–132, 145–147

Inhibitors -microbial 20, 101–102

Interactions
-microbial 19–23, 101–104, 105–107
-enzyme 56, 58, 121
-protein-protein 55
-synergistic 52–53, 183, 187, 190–191

Intron 139–149

Isobutyric acid 30

Isoforms, enzyme 129

Isotricha 69–73

Laccaria amethystina (fucose) lectin (LAF) 169, 172–173

Lachnospira multiparus 16, 103

Lactaria deliciosus lectin (LDL) 169, 172–174, 177

Lactate 102, 179–185, 190, 197, 211–212

Lactate dehydrogenase 180, 187–188, 211

Land use 2–3

Lectins,
-binding to anaerobic fungi 169–174
-carbohydrate specificities 169
-class I, class II definition 167
-taxonomic implications of binding 174–175

Legumes 16

Lespedeza cuneata 15

Lignin 17, 29, 31–32, 34, 38, 73–74, 114
-amount in forage cell walls 9
-and digestibility 17, 31–32, 34
-carbohydrate complexes 21

Localisation, enzyme 53–55, 119–121, 131–132

Lolium perenne 103

Lucerne *(Alfalfa)* 2, 4, 73, 76, 98
-chemical composition 8

Maize 2, 4
-phenolic acids in 34–42
-recombinant inbreds lines 32–42

Malate 179, 180–184, 190–191, 195, 197, 209–212

Malate dehydrogenase 180, 211

Malic enzyme 180, 185–187, 197, 211

Megasphaera elsdenii 103

Methane 20, 102, 183

Methanobacterium bryantii 183

Methanobrevibacter smithii 183, 187–188, 191

Methanobrevibacter arboriphilus 183

Metronidazole 187–188

Microbody 180, 186, 191, 199–200, 203, 223–231

Mimosine 14

Myrica pensylvanica 15

NAD(P)H:ferredoxin oxidoreductase 180, 185–187, 197, 211

Neocallimastix sp. 179–192, 196–197, 211–212, 215, 223, 226, 229–230

Neocallimastix frontalis 83, 99–108, 115, 119, 128–134, 137-149, 172, 179–192, 196–197

N. hurleyensis 83–88

N. joyonii 83

N. patriciarum 83, 99, 132, 182, 196–197

N. variablis 83, 172

NDF
-degradability 43–47

Nigericin 190

Oats 2, 4

Oilseeds 2, 4

Orpinomyces bovis 83

Orpinomyces joyonii 83, 86, 99–100, 172

Paecilomyces fumosoroseus 153, 161

P. persicinum 155

Particle size 17–19

Passage (of digesta) 17–18

Pectin 51

Pectinase 54, 113, 114

Penicillium aculeatum 160

P. allahabadense 155, 160

P. allii 158

P. atramentosum 158

P. brevicompactum 158

P. charlesii 158
P. charmesinum 158
P. chrysogenum 158
P. crustosum 158
P. decumbens 158
P. dendriticum 160
P. diversum 160
P. erubescens 158
P. erythromellis 154, 160
P. expansum 153
P. frequentans 158
P. funiculosum 160
P. hordei 158
P. ingelheimense 158
P. islandicum 160
P. ochrochloron 154
P. oxalicum 158
P. pinophilum 160
P. purpurogenum 160
P. spinulosum 158
P. thomii 158
P. verruculosum 160
Penicillium cell walls 153–162
PEPcarboxykinase 137–149, 180, 211
  -gene 143–149
  -sequence, amino acid 144
  -sequence, nucleotide 143–144
Peroxisome 199, 224–231
pH,
  -rumen 43–47, 70, 75
  -optimum for enzymes 128–129
  -transmembrane gradient 179, 189
Phenolic acids 29–42
  -analysis of, in rumen fluid 37
  -dehydroxylation 35
  -demethoxylation 35
  -esters 32
  -hydrogenation 35
  -phenolic acid esterases 32, 33, 50, 54,
     113, 114, 116
  -release from plant CW 32
Phenylacetic acid 29, 35, 36–37
Phenylalanine 35
3-Phenylpropionic acid 29, 35–37
Pholiota squarrosa lectin (PSL) 169, 172–175
Phosphofructokinase 180, 184, 187
Pichia pastoris 229–230
Piromonas communis 83, 128–129, 183
Piromyces sp. 113–122

Piromyces communis 83, 99–102, 106, 172
P. dumbonica 83, 172
P. mae 83, 172
P. minutis 83
P. rhizinflata 83, 172
P. spiralis 83
Polyethylene glycol 16
Polyplastron 19, 69–73
Polyvinylpyrrolidine 16
Prevotella ruminicola 52, 53, 58, 59
Production
  -crops and residues 3–5
Protease 113, 114
Protein
  -degradability 43–47
  -interactions 55
Protozoa 19
  -cell wall degradation 69–77
  -see generic names *Dasytricha, Entodinium,
     Epidinium, Isotricha, Polyplastron,
     Psalteriomonas, Trichomonas,
     Tritrichomonas.*
Psalteriomonas lanterna 213–217
Pulses 2, 4
Pyruvate 179, 180–184, 195, 197, 209–
  211
Pyruvate ferredoxin oxidoreductase 180,
  182, 185–187, 197, 211
Pyruvate formate lyase 180, 211
Pyruvate kinase 180, 211

Quercus incana 15

Residues, crop 1–8
Rice 2, 4
Robinia 15
Rumen bacteria
  -numbers 44, 46
  -see species names
Rumen fungi
  -see fungi, anaerobic
Ruminococcus albus 20, 51–55, 58, 59, 101
Ruminococcus flavefaciens 18, 20, 21, 51,
  54–61, 99, 101–102, 106
Ruminomyces elegans 83
Rye 2, 4

Saccharomyces cerevisiae 138, 143, 146, 201,
  230

Season
-effect on rumen 43–47
Selenomonas ruminantium 20–21, 102–103
Silica 17
SKL targeting signal 180, 186, 215, 225–226
Sophoria japonica lectin (SJL) 169, 172–174
Soya-bean agglutinin (SBA) 20, 169, 172–173
Sphaeromonas communis 83, 128–129, 183
Straw, cereal 2, 5, 7
-cell wall composition 7
-chemical composition 7
Streptococcus bovis 20, 103
Succinate 99, 179, 189–190, 197, 211–212
Succinate thiokinase 180, 184, 186, 190, 211–213
Synergistes jonesii 14
Syringic acid 29, 36–37

Talaromyces bacillisporus 160
T. byssochlamydoides 158
T. emersonii 158
T. flavus 154, 160
T. helicus 160
T. macrosporus 160
T. mimosinus 160
T. purpureus 160
T. stipitatus 160
Talaromyces cell walls 153–161
Tannins/tannic acid 15–16
Toxins, plant 14–16

Trichoderma 116, 121
Trichomonas vaginalis 210–215
Trimyema compressum 212
Triticale 2, 4
Tritrichomonas foetus 210
Tyrosine 35

Urease 15
Uronic acids 52

Vaccinium nitidum 15
Valinomycin 190
Vanillic acid 29, 36–37
Vitis rotundifolia 15
Volatile fatty acids
-rumen 43–47, 70, 71

Wheat 2, 4
-straw 76, 115
Wheat-germ agglutinin (WGA) 169, 172–175

Xylan 51, 70–72, 115
Xylanase 50, 57–61, 106, 113, 114–122, 127–134
-genes 57–61, 127–134
β-Xylosidase 50, 106, 113, 114–122, 127–134

Ziziphus 15
Zoospore, fungal 80–87, 104, 181, 185, 196